Advances in Gerontological Nursing

1996
Issues for The 21st Century
Elizabeth A. Swanson, PhD, RN, and
Toni Tripp-Reimer, PhD, RN, FAAN, Editors

1997
Chronic Illness and the Older Adult
Elizabeth A. Swanson, PhD, RN, and
Toni Tripp-Reimer, PhD, RN, FAAN, Editors

Elizabeth A. Swanson, PhD, RN, is an Associate Professor in the College of Nursing at The University of Iowa in Iowa City, Iowa. Dr. Swanson received a BS degree in nursing and an MA degree from The University of Iowa College of Nursing, as well as a PhD degree from the College of Education.

Her work focuses on examining the effects of the nursing interventions of family-staff partnerships on staff, family, and residents with Alzheimer's disease. She is also involved in research projects investigating the impact of individualized music therapy and group music therapy on persons with Alzheimer's disease and dementia.

Toni Tripp-Reimer, RN, PhD, FAAN, is Professor and Associate Dean for Research at The University of Iowa College of Nursing in Iowa City, Iowa. She holds an MS in nursing and an MA and PhD in anthropology from The Ohio State University. She is also Director (or PI) of the NIH-funded Center for Gerontological Nursing Interventions Research (P30), the Institutional NRSA Training Program in Gerontological Nursing Research (T32), and the Iowa-Veterans Affairs Nursing Research Consortium.

She has conducted work concerned with health behaviors of ethnic elderly for the past 18 years through a series of seven funded projects. Her current work focuses on issues of medication self-care for rural elders, psychosocial issues in relocation, and assessment and management of acute confusion.

Advances in Gerontological Nursing

Chronic Illness and the Older Adult

Elizabeth A. Swanson, PhD, RN
Toni Tripp-Reimer, PhD, RN, FAAN
Editors

Springer Publishing Company

Springer Publishing Company, Inc.
536 Broadway
New York, NY 10012-3955

Cover design by: Margaret Dunin
Acquisitions Editor: Ruth Chasek
Production Editor: Kathleen Kelly

97 98 99 00 01/5 4 3 2 1

ISBN 0-8261-9111-8
ISSN 1083-8708

Printed in the United States of America

To

Woodrow W. and Inabelle H. Morris

for their contributions to the field of gerontology,

particularly their inspiring support of gerontological nursing research.

Contents

Contributors

Marci Catanzaro, PhD, RN, CS
Gerontological Nurse Practitioner
Primary Health Care Associates
Seattle, Washington 98125
e-mail: catanzar@u.washington.edu

Julie Cheitlin Cherry, RN, BS
Cardiac Staff Nurse
Columbia Homecare and Hospice
San Jose, California
e-mail: medicrbc@ix.netcom.com

Juliet M. Corbin, RN, DNSc, FNP
Lecturer
School of Nursing
San Jose State University
San Jose, California 95192-0057
e-mail: corbin@scruznet.com

Cheryl A. Dellasega, GNP, PhD
Associate Professor
School of Nursing and Department of Biobehavioral Health
The Pennsylvania State University
University Park, Pennsylvania 16802
e-mail: cxd6@email.psu.edu

Margaret Dimond, PhD, RN, FAAN
Professor
School of Nursing
University of Washington
Seattle, Washington 98195-7266
e-mail: dimond@u.washington.edu

Keela A. Herr, PhD, RN, CS
Associate Professor
College of Nursing
The University of Iowa
Iowa City, Iowa 52242
e-mail: keela-herr@uiowa.edu

Margarethe Lorensen, PhD, RN
Institute of Nursing Science
University of Oslo
N-0317 Oslo, Norway
e-mail: margarethe.lorensen@sykepleievit.uio.no

Paula R. Mobily, PhD, RN
Associate Professor
College of Nursing
The University of Iowa
Iowa City, Iowa 52242
e-mail: paula-mobily@uiowa.edu

Janice M. Morse, RN, PhD, FAAN
Professor
School of Nursing
The Pennsylvania State University
University Park, Pennsylvania 16802
e-mail: jmm17@psuvm.psu.edu

Bethel A. Powers, RN, PhD
Associate Professor
School of Nursing
University of Rochester
Rochester, New York 14642
e-mail: powb@son.rochester.edu

Marilyn J. Rantz, PhD, RN
Assistant Professor
University of Missouri-Columbia
School of Nursing
Columbia, Missouri 65211
e-mail: nursrant@showme.missouri.edu

Joanne S. Stevenson, PhD, RN, FAAN
Professor Emeritus
College of Nursing
The Ohio State University
Columbus, Ohio 43210-1289
e-mail: stevenson.3@osu.edu

Elizabeth A. Swanson, PhD, RN
Associate Professor
College of Nursing
The University of Iowa
Iowa City, Iowa 52242
e-mail: elizabeth-swanson@uiowa.edu

Toni Tripp-Reimer, PhD, RN, FAAN
Professor and Associate Dean for Research
College of Nursing
The University of Iowa
Iowa City, Iowa 52242
e-mail: toni-reimer@uiowa.edu

Mary Zwygart-Stauffacher, PhD, RN, CS, GNP
Assistant Professor
University of Minnesota
School of Nursing
Minneapolis, MN 55455
e-mail: zwyga001@tc.umn.edu

National Advisory Panel

Ivo L. Abraham, PhD, CS, RN, FAAN
Professor
Schools of Nursing and Medicine
Charlottesville, Virginia 22903
and
Catholic University of Leuven
Leuven, Belgium

Patricia G. Archbold, RN, DNSc, FAAN
Professor
School of Nursing
Oregon Health Sciences University
Portland, Oregon 97201

Cornelia M. Beck, PhD, RN, FAAN
Professor and Associate Dean for Research and Evaluation
College of Nursing
University of Arkansas for Medical Sciences
Little Rock, Arkansas 72205

Barbara A. Given, PhD, RN, FAAN
Professor and Director of Research
College of Nursing
Michigan State University
East Lansing, Michigan 48824

Virgene Kayser-Jones, PhD, RN, FAAN
Professor
School of Nursing
University of California-San Francisco
San Francisco, California 94143

Kathleen A. McCormick, PhD, RN, FAAN
Senior Science Advisor
Office of Science and Data Development
Agency for Health Care Policy and Research
Rockville, Maryland 20852

Virginia J. Neelon, PhD, RN
Associate Professor and Director
Biobehavioral Laboratory
School of Nursing
The University of North Carolina at Chapel Hill
Chapel Hill, North Carolina 27599

Linda R. Phillips, PhD, RN, FAAN
Professor
College of Nursing
University of Arizona
Tucson, Arizona 85721

Neville E. Strumpf, PhD, RN, C, FAAN
Associate Professor
School of Nursing
University of Pennsylvania
Philadelphia, Pennsylvania 19104

Thelma J. Wells, PhD, RN, FAAN, FRCN
Professor
School of Nursing
University of Wisconsin
Madison, Wisconsin 53792

May L. Wykle, PhD, RN, FAAN
Florence Cellar Professor and Chairperson of Gerontological Nursing
FPB School of Nursing
Case Western Reserve University
Cleveland, Ohio 44106

Introduction

This volume is the second in our series on *Advances in Gerontological Nursing.* In our premier issue, we took the broad view. With an eye toward what we anticipate will be major issues in the 21st century, we offered the Iowa conceptual model of what gerontological nursing is and how it promotes health, provides care, and facilitates transitions for older adults. We reported on several innovative research areas that suggest how gerontological nursing might respond to the specific health needs of older adults of various ethnic backgrounds, to older adults who live in rural settings, to those who are homeless, and to those with cognitive impairments. We considered the role of families providing care for their elderly members and issues related to interventions with those families, and we made some predictions about how the changing demographics of the elderly population in the United States are likely to affect the institutions of care: long-term institutional, community, and home based care.

In this second volume, we shift our vision from the panoramic to the specific and focus intently on a single issue: the care of chronically ill elders.

As all of us in the health professions are keenly aware, people are living longer. They are experiencing chronic illness, the incidence of which tends to increase with age, as well as physiological and sociological changes that can put them at greater risk for not being able to secure the resources they need to manage their health conditions. Thus the recent dramatic increases in the number of older Americans have meant corresponding increases in the number of individuals succumbing to fatal conditions or experiencing nonfatal but permanently debilitating conditions. Along with the higher incidence of chronic illness among older adults has come an increase in the complexity of care and the need for expanded systems of support, as elders may experience several chronic conditions simultaneously and as their capacity to perform daily activities of living changes, often becoming limited in various ways.

Fortunately, as this volume reveals, nursing's knowledge base about the issues related to chronic illness in older adults is rapidly growing, and our approach to the care of chronically ill elders is undergoing tremendous change as we learn to view the enduring nature of long-term disease—whether physical or mental—in the wider context of quality of life and expanded definitions of health and well-being.

In the first chapter, Dimond, Catanzaro, and Lorenson help establish an enlarged perspective as they describe how social, political, and economic factors profoundly influence the quality of care delivered to older adults with chronic illness; how those factors often serve to circumscribe the opportunities for well-being; and how they affect the delivery of certain health care services. In the second chapter, Stevenson promotes a similarly broad viewpoint, one based on a holistic definition of health, and encourages us to look beyond an individual's presenting chronic illness to the greater, non-ill aspect of the person, which remains resilient, full of life, and deserving of attention and support.

Echoes of Stevenson's holistic definition of health and health promotion activities resonate in Chapter 3, as Corbin and Cherry share their research findings regarding how nurses and other health care professionals can assist older persons with chronic health conditions to manage those conditions at home for as long as possible. After describing the Corbin and Strauss Chronic Illness Trajectory Framework, the authors offer a fascinating case study of how the framework was used at a community-based, nurse-managed clinic to help elders living at home enhance their quality of life despite aging and illness.

In Chapter 4, Herr and Mobily draw our attention to the issue of chronic pain in older adults and its multidimensional impact (physical, psychological, social, and spiritual). Examining key barriers to the assessment and management of chronic pain in elders, the authors identify several specific areas requiring systematic investigation and highlight the value of integrating multidimensional strategies to manage chronic pain in elders and improve their functional ability, general mood, and overall quality of life.

Although nursing's understanding of the significance of ethnicity and its impact on care issues is growing, there has been little systematic examination of the highly dynamic interrelationship among ethnicity, aging, and chronic illness. Tripp-Reimer delves into this analysis in Chapter 5, presenting demographic data on ethnic populations, describing the health status and distribution of chronic illnesses among those groups, and delineating how the distinctive life patterns that characterize an ethnic group contribute to variations in health behavior as well as different systems of formal and informal care.

One aspect of chronic illness commonly experienced by many older persons is the likelihood that the chronic condition over time will diminish the person's independent functioning and mobility. This functional impairment contributes to increased isolation and a sense of loneliness even as it increases that person's needs for supportive interaction with a network of family, friends, and helpful agencies or institutions. In Chapter 6, Powers places the issue of chronic illness in elders in the context of social support, social networks, and the problem of loneliness. After reviewing the research on social support and social networks, especially as it pertains to particularly vulnerable older adults, she considers the conceptual and methodological limitations of that research and argues for more research specifically focused on elders' experience of loneliness.

While quantitative research on chronic illness in elders informs much of the work presented in the previous chapters, Chapter 7 provides a glimpse into how qualitative research can contribute to a richer, more comprehensive understanding of what it is like to be old, to live with functional impairments, and to cope with the knowledge that complete recovery is not possible. Morse and Dellasega not only describe the process of qualitative research and recommend specific methodological modifications to adapt the process to elderly subjects, they ably demonstrate how qualitative descriptions can be used to explore the experience of chronically ill elders, the impact of their context of care, and the development of theories and specific strategies of care that can lead to improved quality of life.

As Rantz and Zwygart-Stauffacher explain in Chapter 8, institutions providing long-term care to residents who are chronically ill are major players in the health care delivery system. Concerns about quality of care in those institutions have gradually given rise to a host of government policies and regulations regarding the delivery of service. The authors report the findings of their descriptive study designed to identify the major institutional policy related to the care of the chronically ill and discuss the role of professional nurses in influencing and shaping policy decisions before they are made as well as implementing them after they are made.

In addition to the singular topic of this volume, which reflects our desire to expand nursing's knowledge base about chronic illness and the older adult, there is another thread underlying and unifying the disparate chapters: an emerging realization of the need for accessible health care for this population group and of nursing's role in ensuring that need is met. In the epilogue, Swanson elaborates on this overarching theme, indicating how each of the chapters touch on it from their unique perspectives, and how their ideas find support in several government reports. As she describes the development of a range of long-term care service choices and alternatives, she identifies some of the policy issues that would hinder or support their development. Again, the role of the nurse in helping not only to implement but also to set these policies is evident.

This volume, then, can be considered a clarion call not just to a broader vision of a single topic, but also to a wider scope of action related to that topic. It remains critically important for us to continue pursuing research that will expand our understanding of the relationship between age and chronic illness; improve our means of assessing and managing chronic illness and chronic pain; promote a view of health that focuses on the entire individual and not just on a chronic condition; increase our understanding of the relationships among ethnicity, aging, and chronic illness; facilitate support systems and networks that alleviate loneliness; and so on. Yet we must also take the initiative to catapult from that knowledge base and expand our spheres of influence into those arenas where we can identify and press for enlightened policies. On the shoulders of our expanded knowledge base and our commitment to informed action, nursing could truly help raise the quality of care provided to older adults with chronic illness and elevate the quality of life they experience.

Elizabeth Swanson, PhD, RN
Toni Tripp-Reimer, PhD, RN, FAAN
Co-Editors

Acknowledgments

In feeling fortunate regarding the success of the first volume of *Advances in Gerontological Nursing,* we also found that each volume presents its own set of challenges and opportunities to learn fresh lessons from new friends as well as old. We would therefore like to offer our foremost thanks to the authors who have contributed their knowledge and shared their vision with us in this volume. Individually and collectively, their critical sense of what questions must be asked and their dedication to finding answers enrich these pages. Secondly, we would like to acknowledge the unflagging support exhibited by the gerontological nursing faculty at The University of Iowa and the continued guidance of the National Advisory Panel toward this enterprise; both groups have provided invaluable assistance. We continue to feel fortunate to be working with the expert staff of Dr. Ursula Springer's publishing company, particularly Ruth Chasek, Louise Farkas, and Rose Pintaudi, who have been consistently pleasant, extraordinarily accommodating of hectic schedules, and absolutely dedicated to producing work of high caliber. We also appreciate the many ways in which our program staff member, Mary Anders, with her organizational skills and technical knowledge has considerably lightened our load.

Finally, we are grateful to all the readers who responded so positively to our premier issue and fortified our belief that there is indeed a need for this series.

Acknowledgments

CHAPTER 1

Chronic Illness Issues and the Older Adult

Margaret Dimond, Marci Catanzaro, and Margarethe Lorensen

The aging of the population will be the most significant social phenomenon of the 21st century. Its impact will be increasingly felt in political and economic arenas and consequently in that of health. And the impact will be worldwide. The populations of North America, Latin America, Europe, and Asia are aging at approximately equal rates, due primarily to decreasing fertility and mortality rates. The United Nations (1993) projected that the 65 and older population will number 822 million worldwide by 2025, exceeding the present combined populations of Europe and North America. The proportion of older people in the world's population will increase from 6.2% in 1990 to 9.7% in 2025 (Preston & Martin, 1994). Chronic illness issues and health care for older adults can be expected to increase with the aging of the population (Estes & Rundall, 1992).

The literature contains many definitions of chronic illness. For this chapter, chronic conditions are defined as "long term diseases, injuries with long sequelae, and enduring structural, sensory and communication abnormalities. They are physical or mental (cognitive and emotional), and their onset time ranges from birth to late in life. Their defining aspect is duration. Once they are past certain symptomatic and diagnostic thresholds, chronic conditions are essentially permanent features for the rest of life" (Verbrugge & Patrick, 1995, p. 173). An examination of the issues of health care for older adults with chronic illnesses cannot be done apart from the larger social, political, and economic context within which health care is delivered. Nurses (whether educators, practitioners, or researchers) will need to understand these issues to comprehend fully and work within this larger context for the benefit of older adults.

SOCIAL, POLITICAL, AND ECONOMIC CONTEXT OF HEALTH CARE FOR OLDER ADULTS

The context of health care for older adults, mentioned previously, has a profound impact on the quality of health care for older adults with chronic illnesses. This context can be recognized in the priorities for research funding, the limitations of health care insurance coverage, availability and access to care, and the social structures that determine economic well-being in later life. In this chapter, the manner in which these macrofactors are manifested in the everyday lives of older adults with chronic illnesses are discussed from three perspectives, namely, gender, poverty, and ethnicity. A recent analysis of chronic illness, activity levels, and use of health services provides a background for this discussion.

Using available statistics on seven chronic conditions (three nonfatal: arthritis, visual impairment, hearing impairment, and four fatal: ischemic heart disease, chronic obstructive pulmonary disease, diabetes mellitus, malignant neoplasms), Verbrugge and Patrick (1995) point out three factors important to the understanding of the impact of chronic illness in later years.

1. All seven of the previously named chronic conditions can result in diminished ability to perform roles and participate in valued activities, can increase the use of outpatient services, and may lead to hospitalization for acute medical episodes or surgery.
2. With increased age the nonfatal conditions have a functional limiting impact equivalent to that of the fatal conditions.
3. Even in the face of demonstrated disability and use of health services for chronic conditions, mortality rates still drive the political agenda. That is, research funds are allocated to conditions that cause death and not to conditions that cause morbidity.

In the words of Verbrugge and Patrick (p. 180), "common, nonfatal conditions such as arthritis, hearing and visual impairment, incontinence, bunions, and migraine headaches are less likely to secure research and program funds, a situation scarcely commensurate with their frequency and impact on daily life." The remainder of this chapter will build on the previous analysis and show (1) how the social, political and economic context of health care determines the opportunities for functional well-being of three groups of older adults with chronic health problems: women, the poor, and persons of color, and (2) how the social, political, and economic *context* of health care translates into the *delivery* of care in two types of health service needs for older adults: mental health and rehabilitation. We will argue that nurses need to be informed and to participate in the professional and political debates that will determine future health care priorities for older adults.

Gender Issues

Older women will continue to outnumber men by a margin of three to one worldwide. Given that the world population of older adults is and increasingly will be women, many of whom have chronic conditions, it seems clear that many of the issues of aging and health care are women's issues (Dimond, 1995). That is not to say that older men with chronic illnesses are not or will not be disadvantaged in current health care systems, but only to suggest that women, particularly women of color, are at greater risk in the current sociopolitical and economic context of health care. This greater risk is due, as well, to the fact that although mortality rates for older women are lower than those for older men, women have greater morbidity due to chronic illnesses and more limitations in self-care (Task Force on Older Women's Health, 1993). "Chronic, disabling conditions limit the quality of life for millions of women, particularly elderly women" (*Commonwealth Fund Survey of Women's Health,* 1993, p. 11). For example, 26% of women and 18% of men have been told in the past 5 years that they have arthritis, and 8% of women have been told they have nonskin cancer compared to 3% of men. Urinary incontinence is a serious health and social problem for older women. Eight percent of women and 2% of men have an episode of urinary incontinence during any given week.

The receipt of quality health care for older women with chronic conditions is dependent on several factors, among which are the knowledge and attitudes of health care providers and access to health services. The Task Force on Older Women's Health (1993) reported that physician education needs to include content on older women's health and gender differences in manifestation of disease and response to treatment. This content is needed to overcome biases in diagnosis and treatment of a variety of illnesses, including breast and lung cancer, menopause/osteoporosis, depression, urinary incontinence, and cardiovascular disease. Health care for older women with cardiovascular disease is an example of the need for better training in and sensitivity to women's health. Women undergo intensive or invasive evaluations and treatments for cardiac disease substantially less often than men who experience symptoms of similar or lesser severity; this is particularly true for the evaluation of chest pain (Ayanian & Epstein, 1991; Tobin et al., 1987; Wenger, Speroff, & Packard, 1993). In a longitudinal study of 246 older myocardial infarction (MI) patients, one-third of whom were women, Young and Kahana (1993) found that at 6 weeks post-MI, men had received significantly more information about heart disease than women and were more likely than women to be referred to cardiac rehabilitation programs and diagnostic angiograms. At the 1-year follow-up, women showed less favorable recovery than men. For example, women reported more sick days, more shortness of breath, more angina, and overall greater functional limitations than men. Although the rate of early post-MI death is greater in women than men, it is uncertain whether this excess mortality reflects "the older age, smaller body size, or more frequent and severe coexisting illnesses of women when symptomatic coronary disease occurs, or whether it results from suboptimal or delayed care" (Wenger et al., p. 247). The answers to these unknowns will depend on research funds directed toward investigations of illnesses that are common to women or are manifested in ways that differ from men.

The attitudes of physicians toward women patients were recently documented in a large representative survey on women's health (*Commonwealth Fund Survey of Women's Health,* 1993). The survey was conducted by Louis Harris and Associates, Inc., and included interviews with 2,500 women and 1,000 men from 18 years of age to over 65. Thirty-two percent of women in this survey reported changing their doctors because of communication problems. Women of all ages reported having more difficulties than men in talking with their physicians. Twenty-five percent of women reported that physicians "talked down to them," whereas 12% of men reported this. Seventeen percent of women also reported they were told their conditions were "all in their heads," compared to 7% of men. Quality care for women is significantly jeopardized by communication patterns such as these.

Expert knowledge and skillful, sensitive communication on the part of health care providers are of little value if access to health care is problematic. Access can be defined in physical/environmental terms (e.g., rural/

urban), psychological terms (e.g., communication problems with primary care provider), and economic and political terms (e.g., comprehensive health insurance). Although access to quality care, defined in physical/environmental or psychological terms, is an issue for both older men and women, the focus here is on access defined in economic and political terms, in which case older women are more disadvantaged than older men. Arendell and Estes (1991, p. 59) point out that health care issues facing older women are not a result of old age, but "of lifelong patterns of socioeconomic and gender stratification in the larger society." These authors are quick to point out that the long-term solutions to health care issues for older women cannot be found by simply providing more services, necessary and worthwhile as they may be. Enduring change will only come about when the root causes are addressed. That is, "gender, race, and age discrimination in the labor market, unequal pay for comparable work, quality of income security programs for women, and a lifetime of devalued caregiving work" (Arendell & Estes, p. 60) must be addressed and corrected. The consequences of socioeconomic and political biases based on both gender and race become apparent in an analysis of poverty among older adults.

Poverty, Age, and Health Care

"Income is one of the most important dimensions of social class in predicting health status" (Estes & Rundall, 1992, p. 304). Most studies of income and poverty rates among older adults show that overall income is up and poverty rates are down (Gilford, 1988; Quinn & Smeeding, 1993; U.S. Congress, 1991; U.S. Department of Commerce, 1992). Global and undifferentiated analysis of the economic well-being of older adults will generally show the same trends, but undifferentiated analysis of income and poverty rates is inappropriate given the heterogeneity of the aging population (Quinn, 1987; Radner, 1992). There is wide variation in poverty rates among older adults. For example, the oldest-old (the most rapidly growing segment of this population) are most likely to be poor. The poverty rates for older African Americans and Hispanics are two to three times higher than for non-Hispanic whites (Taeuber, 1992). Among all older women, poverty rates for non-Hispanic, Hispanic, and African American older women are widely divergent (13%, 25%, and 39%, respectively) (U.S. Department of Commerce). These rates are even more dramatic when women live alone. Fifty percent of older Hispanic women and nearly 60% of older African American women who live alone are poor.

The largest single source of financial income for older adults is Social Security (nearly 40%), followed by earnings, property income, and private and public pensions. Noncash benefits (Medicare, Medicaid, food stamps, and subsidized housing) account for about 10% of total income (Gilford, 1988). Adult women, regardless of race or ethnicity, urban or rural residence, age or labor force participation, are more likely than adult men to be poor (Perales, 1988). As noted previously, Arendell and Estes (1991) have argued this fact specifically for older women. More recently, Burkhauser (1994, p. 148) noted that "despite massive social security expenditures, older women remain the most vulnerable members of our society, in part because of a substantial drop in the level of social security protection they receive following the death of their spouse." As long as Social Security is based on years of continuous participation in the labor force, older women will continue to have a disadvantaged economic status.

Of all noncash benefits for older adults, Medicare and Medicaid are the largest sources. For many, these sources of health care financing have been of incalculable value. But here, as in the Social Security system, women are at greater risk than men. Most of the morbidity of older women is due to chronic conditions, such as arthritis, hypertension, osteoporosis and its sequelae, dementia, depression, urinary incontinence, vision, hearing, and foot problems. Although these conditions may at times require hospitalization, the major source of health care is community-based. And herein lies the problem. Medicare is heavily weighted toward acute services and high-technology medical care and thus provides limited coverage for the common chronic conditions of older women. This accounts for the fact that older women currently spend as much on health care (about 15% of their income) as they did prior to the passage of Medicare in 1965 (Prospective Payment Assessment Commission, 1989). Medicare covers such costs as hospitals, skilled nursing and rehabilitation services, skilled home health services, physician cost (and in some cases nurse practitioners), and laboratory costs incurred on an outpatient basis. However, there are numerous exceptions, copayments, deductibles, stringent limitations on the length of time covered services can be provided, and other requirements that place considerable limitations on reimbursement. Medicare does not cover, or covers in extremely limited ways, many important health care services required by older adults, such as long-term care in nursing homes (in which women are overrepresented), medications prescribed for outpatients, hearing aids, eyeglasses, dentures, preventive health examinations, rehabilitation services, and outpatient psychotherapy. In an analysis of Medicare reimbursement differences by gender, Sofaer and Abel (1990) have shown that after taking Medicare reimbursement into account, three of four illnesses with high out-of-pocket costs (hypertension, arthritis, and depression) are more common among women than among men. The fourth high out-of-pocket condition, stroke, is not gender-related. Hypertension, arthritis, and depression are chronic conditions that require regular monitoring by a physician, and thus frequent use of medical services and continuing out-of-pocket costs for older women. Similar results can be found in reports of Medicaid coverage for the poor. Among older men and women, women represent 62% of those eligible for Medicaid. Thus Medicaid coverage is both a class and gender issue, since more older women than men are likely to be poor (Muller, 1988). Being old, female and poor is sometimes referred to as "triple jeopardy." But the consequences of age, gender, and economic status are further compounded by ethnicity.

Issues of Ethnicity

Issues of particular significance for ethnically diverse older persons with chronic illnesses are poverty, advocacy and access to health services and appropriate use of these services, heterogeneity within ethnic groups, and so-called color-blind approaches to health care (Frank-Stromberg, 1991; Hopper, 1993; Johnson, 1994; McKenna, 1989; Yee, 1992).

Poverty is almost endemic in some minority groups and its consequences are fairly well known. For example, poor African Americans over the age of 65 are twice as likely as non-Hispanic whites to lack health insurance (whether Medicare, Medicaid, or aid from the Veteran's Administration, VA) (Ries, 1987). Similarly, low-income African Americans have fewer physician contacts, fewer short-stay hospitalizations, more serious acute episodes, and more restricted activity days per person than comparably poor white older adults (National Center for Health Statistics, 1990). Although data for other minority groups, such as Hispanics, Pacific Islanders, Asian Americans, and Native Americans, are marginally available and inconsistent, there is a trend toward more acute and disabling conditions, similar to those found among older poor African Americans (Yee, 1992). Distinctions need to be made between the chronic poor and those who become poor with the death of a spouse (usually women). Most of the efforts to reverse poverty levels of older adults have been to "prevent" poverty, that is, to employ strategies to assist those who become poor in later life. Few efforts have been directed toward reducing poverty and increasing access to health care for elders who have lived in poverty all their lives (Yee).

Poor access to health care for chronically ill and poor older adults of color is due to a variety of situations. Lack of knowledge of health care resources and how to "work" the health care system, lack of insurance and knowledge of how to acquire the insurance to which they have a right, unavailable health services or poor transportation to available services, and perceived (and often real) discrimination are the major reasons for poor access to health care by poor older adults of color (Yeatts, Crow, & Folts, 1992).

There seems to be a widely held assumption that all people of color who belong to the same race hold the same values and health beliefs and practice the same health behavior. There is often a failure on the part of health care providers to recognize that "ethnicity is not merely a set of artifacts and labels, language or dress, but rather a fluid concept that changes and adapts over time, changes among generations, and often re-emerges in later life as an integrating force in the transition to age, providing a sense of continuity of self and community" (Gelfand & Baressi, 1987, p. 5). This cultural insensitivity is widespread even though the literature on aging and ethnicity is repetitive in its insistence on the need to acknowledge the heterogeneity of ethnic populations, indeed of all older adults. One consequence of this insensitivity is a type of care sometimes referred to as "color-blind care." Although this term was intended to convey a certain equality of care for all people, it actually presents a formidable barrier to care. Color-blind care may result in inadequate or inappropriate care since values, beliefs, customs, and language diversity are not integrated into a plan of care.

Summary

Older adults who have chronic illnesses face many challenges as they learn to live with a compromised health status. These challenges are particularly difficult for women, those who are poor, and those who belong to ethnic groups of color. Health care for older adults is firmly entrenched in a system that is biased against women, the poor, and people of color. It is within the context of this system that health care is delivered to older adults. The next section describes how the delivery of health care for chronically ill older adults is determined by this context.

DELIVERY OF CARE TO CHRONICALLY ILL OLDER ADULTS

The delivery of clinical services to older adults with chronic illnesses and limitations in functional performance occurs within the social, cultural, economic, and political context outlined previously. The impact of this context on the delivery of health care to chronically ill or functionally compromised older adults is discussed in this section for two specific areas of health care: mental health and conditions that require rehabilitation. These two areas were selected for four reasons:

1. Both, if neglected, have a profound impact on the functional ability of older adults;
2. Both have been more neglected by researchers than conditions viewed as more likely to be funded, that is, they do not fit the national political agenda (Verbrugge & Patrick, 1995);
3. Both have limited public visibility, as they do not attract print or television media coverage; and
4. Each is stigmatized, either by the misplaced belief that it is somehow a blemish of character (mental illness) or it is not responsive to treatment and is therefore unnecessary (conditions requiring rehabilitation).

Mental Health Issues

Overall, mental health care for older adults receives less attention than physical health in health professions' curricula, the federal research agenda, or third-party reimbursement policies. An exception to this is Alzheimer's Disease and other dementias. Yet one of the most frequent psychogeriatric disorders of older adulthood is *depression,* and the rate of suicide (a potential consequence of depression) has increased steadily in this population over the past decade (National Center for Health Statistics, 1988). Similarly, the risks and consequences of *alcohol dependency* in the aged are very poorly understood; yet alcohol dependency accounts for considerable morbidity and cost, and may be associated with depression (Atkinson, 1990; Brennan, Moos, & Kim, 1993). These are major chronic illness concerns for older adults.

In the developed countries, about one-quarter of those aged 65 and over suffer from mental disorders (Hafner & Weyerer, 1986). Risk factors for mental illnesses in this population are numerous and often unavoidable. Among these are deficits in social relationships and perceived loneliness, conjugal bereavement, diminished physical capacity with attendant functional limitations, low self-esteem, and diminished personal control. Mental illness among older adults is compounded by the low utilization of outpatient mental health services (often due to stigma or financial circumstances). Depression and alcohol problems are likely to be underdiagnosed and undertreated in older adults, in part because the present health care system discriminates against women, the poor, and people of color.

Depression

Depression among older adults is less common than at other ages, but the prevalence of significant dysphoria is considerable. Blazer, Hughes, and George (1987) found less than 1% of community-dwelling older adults had a major depressive disorder, but over 26% experienced significant dysphoria. Although the reported prevalence of depressive disorders in older adults may vary significantly due to the diagnostic criteria used to establish prevalence, most epidemiologic findings show that depressive disorders in older adults are far too frequent to be ignored (Anthony & Aboraya, 1992). Depression may be masked by hypochondriasis or somatization (Casey, 1994), thus increasing the possibility of missed or inaccurate diagnosis. Concomitant factors such as immobility, few social and financial resources, and self-neglect caused by depression may exacerbate coexisting chronic illnesses and frailty (Rabins, 1992). There are a number of risk factors for major depressive disorders and dysthymia. Being female is a significant factor until about age 80, when prevalence among males surpasses females (Gurland, Dean, Cross, & Golden, 1980). Other risk factors are inadequate level or type of social support (Goldberg, Van Natta, & Comstock, 1985), previous depressive illness episodes (Koenig & Blazer, 1992), and loss of a spouse (Dimond, Caserta, & Lund, 1994). Physical health status, such as number of chronic illnesses, self-perceived health, physician visits, and number of prescribed medications, has consistently been associated with depressed affect (Koenig & Blazer). For older adults who have suffered a stroke, the rate of depression was 43% in men and 64% in women (Murrell, Himmelfarb, & Wright, 1983). Of more importance than the diagnostic category of a chronic illness is the severity of the condition and the extent of functional disability that accompanies it. Callahan, Hui, Nienaber, Musick, and Tierney (1994) reported that community-dwelling older adults with significant depressive symptoms were more likely to rate their health as fair or poor, use more emergency room and outpatient visits, and incur higher outpatient charges (due to the limited reimbursement of mental health services) than older adults who were not depressed.

The data on depression among older persons of color are sparse and sometimes contradictory. Stanford and Du Bois (1992) summarized the existing knowledge under the broad framework of mental health problems and ethnicity. Briefly, among African Americans the prevalence of depression is 23%, and is largely associated with poor financial resources, reduced social network contact, and inadequate caregiver support. Epidemiologic data for Hispanic American elders, Native Americans, and Asian Pacific Islanders are extremely sparse. The data that are available show that Hispanic women are more likely to be depressed than Hispanic men (Morton, Schoenrock, Stanford, Peddecord, & Molgaard, 1989). In a large epidemiologic study conducted in Los Angeles, 71% of all depressed Hispanic elders were women (Kemp, Staples, & López-Aqueres, 1987). Most of the depressed subjects were non-English speaking, with less than 5 years of formal education, widowed, and with annual incomes below $6,000. Hispanic elders underutilize health services, including mental health services, due in part to the absence of bilingual and bicultural services. Among Native Americans the use of the Indian Health Services (IHS) for mental health is lowest among those who are over 65 years of age. Korean Americans have higher overall depression scores than any other Asian group, but they underutilize mental health services. As in the case of Hispanic elderly, an underlying factor in the utilization of mental health services by Korean Americans is the absence of culturally sensitive services (Stanford & Du Bois). Taken as a whole, risk factors for mental health problems among all persons of color are high stress and a lifetime of lower earning potential, which translates into fewer coping resources.

Evidence for depression in institutionalized older adults (70%–80% of whom are women) is less clear than that for community-dwelling elders. Nonetheless, the existing evidence suggests that depression is common among institutionalized older adults (Parmelee, Katz, & Lawton, 1989). In a recent document addressing barriers to mental health care in nursing homes, Lombardo (1994) stated that approximately 65% of the 1.6 million nursing home residents in the United States have mental disorders, a significant type being depression, which is often comorbid with dementia. Additional studies show that major depressive disorders affect 12%–18% of nursing home residents and an additional 30%–35% have other depressive disorders (Parmalee et al., 1989; Weissman, Bruce, Leaf, Florio, & Holzer, 1991). Koenig and Blazer (1992) note that after cognitive impairments, depressive illness is the most common psychiatric disorder in the institutionalized aged, and clearly the most reversible.

Recognition and treatment of depression among older community-dwelling adults by primary care physicians is very low. Yet these are the providers most likely to have the opportunity to identify depression in this population. Rapp and Davis (1989) reported that medical residents considered the identification and treatment of comorbid depression to be important, but knew little about the diagnostic criteria, rarely screened for depression, and generally believed that treatment for depression in older adults was ineffective. Recognition and treatment of depressed residents in nursing homes is similarly inadequate. Heston et al. (1992) reported that of 868 nursing home residents diagnosed with depression, only 10% were treated with antidepressants. Benzodiazepines or neuroleptics were more often prescribed for depression than antidepressants. In 52% of the cases of diagnosed depression, no psychoactive drugs were prescribed. These authors concluded that even when a diagnosis of depression is made and recorded, most nursing home residents remain untreated, incorrectly treated, or inadequately treated. Lombardo (1994, p. 1) summarized the failure to treat depression in nursing homes as follows:

> Shortages of mental health professionals trained in geriatrics, lack of training of nursing home personnel, the inappropriate use of psychotropic drugs and physical restraints, poor linkages between mental health providers and nursing homes, and restrictive Medicare and Medicaid reimbursement policies all act as barriers to appropriate treatment and oversight.

The most devastating potential consequence of depression is suicide. Cross-sectional epidemiologic studies show that older adults have the highest suicide rate of any age group (National Center for Health Statistics, 1986). Although older adults constitute nearly 13% of the U.S. population, they account for 17%–25% of reported suicides annually. In 1985, the suicide rate for the general population was 12.3 per 100,000 per year; it was double for individuals 75 to 84 years of age and greater than 56 per 100,000 for white males over 85 years of age (National Center for Health Statistics). Additional data from the National Center for Health Statistics (1988) showed that the rate of suicide among older adults has increased steadily from 17.1 per 100,000 in 1981 to 21.5 per 100,000 in 1986. Precipitation of suicide among older adults has been shown to relate to family discord, financial problems, physical or psychiatric illness, alcoholism, loss, isolation, and hopelessness (Conwell, Rotenberg, & Caine, 1990; Hill, Gallagher, Thompson, & Ishida, 1988). With increasing age, physical illness becomes a predominant precipitant (Conwell et al.). A disturbing finding in the study by these investigators of older adult suicides included 53 subjects with documented psychiatric contacts. Of these, 13 victims of suicide (24.5%) had last seen a therapist within 1 week of death, and an additional 7 (13.2%) had contact within the last month of life (Conwell et al., p. 642).

Many of the issues of depression, suicide, and chronic illness among older adults, both community-dwelling and institutionalized, remain unclear and need further research. For example, there is very little empirical data on the relationship between people of color and whites and mental illness, and between rural and urban dwellers and mental illness. A recent publication by Abraham, Buckwalter, Neese, and Fox (1994) begins to identify mental health issues of older adults who reside in rural settings and to suggest important areas for nursing research.

Alcohol Dependence

The National Institute on Alcohol Abuse and Alcoholism estimates that between 2% and 10% of individuals over the age of 60 suffer from alcoholism (Dufour, Archer, & Gordis, 1992). Awareness of alcohol problems among older adults is increasing, but often remains undetected or ignored by health care providers. "Clinical features, social factors, and professional biases contribute to under-recognition, under-reporting, and under-referral" (Atkinson, Ganzini, & Bernstein, 1992, p. 519). In addition, the absence of a standardized terminology in the identification and reporting of alcohol problems may also contribute to underreporting and underreferral. The term "alcohol dependence" or "alcohol problems" is used here to refer to a wide variety of types of alcohol problems reported in the literature, including alcoholism, alcohol abuse, and alcohol misuse. Older adults with alcohol problems often enter the health care system with problems other than dependence on alcohol, even though the presenting health problems are a consequence of or related to alcohol or medication misuse. Presenting symptoms are often subtle, or atypical, and can be confused with other conditions common to older adults. It is not uncommon for older adults to present alcohol problems as medical or social complaints, or as global emotional issues rather than as alcoholism or drinking concerns

(Burns, 1994). Older female problem drinkers are especially likely to conceal the presentation of alcohol problems with symptoms of depression and reliance on psychoactive drugs (Brennan, Moos, & Kim, 1993). Regardless of age, women are less likely than men to have their alcohol problems diagnosed (Blume, 1990). Studies of the use of emergency medical services by persons with alcohol problems have rarely included older adults. An exception to this was a study to determine the prevalence of alcohol dependence among older adults using the emergency room (ER) for care, in which it was shown that physicians detected only 21% of the concurrent alcohol dependence (Adams, Magruder-Habib, Trued, & Broome, 1992). The prevalence rate of ER use in this study was 14%, with gastrointestinal symptoms being the most common presenting complaint.

The financial cost to the health care system of alcohol dependence is substantial. Adams, Yuan, Barboriak, and Rimm (1993) found that the prevalence of alcohol-related hospitalizations among people aged 65 and older in 1989 was 54.7 per 10,000 population for men and 14.8 per 10,000 for women. There was considerable geographic variation in this national survey, with prevalence ranging from 18.9 per 10,000 in Arkansas to 77.0 per 10,000 in Alaska. The hospitalization charges to Medicare for all admissions (n = 33,039) in which the primary diagnosis was alcohol related totaled $233,543,500, with the median charge per hospital stay of $4,514. In an analysis of alcohol-related diagnosis (ARD), utilization rates by Native Americans and Alaska Natives (NA/AN) in 43 hospitals of the IHS, Hisnanick and Erickson (1993) estimated the total annual utilization rate at 13.7%. These investigators also estimated how much of the hospital inpatient resources had been used for ARD hospitalizations. In IHS hospitals of 50 beds or fewer (which includes three-fourths of all IHS hospitals), 25% of resources were used for ARD hospitalizations. The VA health care system treats a high proportion of older adults and minorities with alcohol dependency problems. In 1985, the costs of care for alcohol dependency and abuse in the VA was $188 million (Rice, Kelman, Miller, & Dunmeyer, 1990). The cost to the federal and state governments for treatment of alcohol problems, whether through Medicare, Medicaid, the VA, or the IHS, is substantial.

While the relative level of alcohol use among older adults is lower than for other age groups, the potential for development of problem drinking is comparatively high because of physiological changes that alter and increase the physiological effects of alcohol. The national prevalence rates of alcohol dependence in community-dwelling older adults, as determined by the Epidemiologic Catchment Area (ECA) study, using the *Diagnostic and Statistical Manual of Mental Disorders,* 3rd ed., revised (DSM-III-R) criteria, showed that the prevalence rate for males 65 years and over was 14%, and for women the corresponding prevalence rate was 1.5% (Robins, Helzer, Przybeck, & Reigier, 1988). The relatively low alcohol problem prevalence at the present time suggests that for today's seniors, alcohol problems are at least partly a cohort effect (e.g., historical experiences such as the Prohibition Era of 1920–33), rather than a period effect (e.g., developments in clinical practice and research, and greater awareness of the problem). Although alcohol dependence is a disorder characterized by male predominance, there is substantial evidence that the prevalence rates for young women are increasing dramatically, especially among young women aged 18–29, where currently these rates are 7%. This statistic is considerably higher than the current rate for women over age 65 (1.5%) and does not bode well for future cohorts of older women (Cloninger, Bohman, & Sigvardsson, 1981; Cloninger, Reich, Sigvardsson, Von Knoring, & Bohman, 1987). Alcohol problems are a significant factor in chronic illness among older men and an emerging significant problem for older women.

An important issue in determining the extent and severity of alcohol problems is caused by widely varying definitions and criteria for diagnosis, and the absence of valid and reliable screening instruments for research or clinical practice. Present screening and diagnostic methods for alcohol use disorders lack adequate validation for older persons (Atkinson, 1990). The *Diagnostic and Statistical Manual of Mental Disorders,* 4th ed. (American Psychiatric Association, 1994), which distinguishes between alcohol abuse and alcohol dependence, is a reasonable guide, but no studies have been done to determine the validity for older adults. In fact, the DSM-IV criteria are difficult to apply to older adults since the diagnostic emphasis is on the consequences of alcohol use. Older adults do not have the same vulnerability as younger adults for the development of the consequences outlined by these standardized criteria. For instance, they are frequently no longer employed, they live alone or apart from family and thus have minimal work or family obligations, and most do not experience significant legal problems as a result of their alcohol use since many no longer operate a motor vehicle. The major consequences of alcohol use among older adults are psychiatric and medical problems (Miller, Belkin, & Gold, 1991), neither of which are identified by the DSM-IV criteria as consequences of alcohol use.

A major risk factor for older adults who are problem users of alcohol is the high number and types of medications they commonly use. The elderly receive from 25% to 30% of all prescriptions, and the average older person uses between two and seven prescription and proprietary medicines a year, as much as two and one-half times the use rate of other age groups (Lawson & Lawson, 1993). Seniors are also heavy users of proprietary or over-the-counter (OTC) medications. It is estimated that 34% of individuals over 60 years of age use OTC drugs (Dufour et al., 1992). The concomitant use of alcohol and OTC drugs increases the risk for many other types of health problems for this age group.

Risk factors for alcohol dependency among older adults are not widely discussed in the literature, perhaps because comparatively few studies of older adults and alcohol use have been done. Differences in alcohol dependency by gender have received somewhat more attention than differences by ethnic group or socioeconomic status. There is beginning evidence to support the impact of life stressors on alcohol use by older adults. Increasingly, investigators are distinguishing between antecedent and consequent factors in late onset versus early onset of alcohol problems in older adults. Late onset is identified by the onset of alcohol problems after age 60 (Atkinson, 1994), or after age 50 (Schonfeld & Dupree, 1991). Atkinson reports that as many as 25%–66% of older adults in treatment for alcohol problems had onset after age 60.

Women are more at risk than men to become alcohol dependent in later life (Atkinson, 1990; Holzer et al., 1984). Older adults with early-onset alcohol dependency are more likely to be known to health care providers and have long-standing health problems similar to young adult problem drinkers. Late-onset alcohol dependency is less likely to be diagnosed as such and therefore less likely to be treated appropriately. Late-middle-aged women with drinking problems (time of onset not reported) have been found to use more psychoactive medication, to be more depressed, and to be less likely to seek treatment for alcohol problems than their male counterparts (Brennan et al., 1993).

Very limited data are available to estimate the risk of alcohol use by ethnic group, or by age and ethnic group membership, but what information is available shows overall greater risks for ethnic minorities. Elevated mortality rates from alcohol use among Native Americans is well established (Heath, 1989); Hispanic men have higher prevalence rates for alcohol-related disorders than either Caucasians or African Americans (Caetano, 1989); and African Americans have higher rates of abstinence, but significantly higher mortality rates from cirrhosis than Caucasians (Herd, 1990). Booth, Blow, Cook, Bunn, and Fortney (1992, p. 1029), in their study of age and ethnicity among hospitalized alcoholics, found that persons of color were significantly younger than Caucasian alcoholics. Hispanics and African Americans, as well as older alcoholics, were less likely to complete treatment or attend detoxification and more likely to be hospitalized for other primary diagnoses. Native Americans, however, were most likely to complete alcoholism treatment. Race and ethnicity have not received adequate attention in the study of late-onset alcohol problems (Atkinson, 1994).

Serious chronic physical illness, social isolation, lack of formal or informal support systems, environmental and social stress, difficulty with personal care and activities of daily living, significant cognitive impairment, and depression are risk factors contributing to alcohol problems among older adults. Fear of loss of independence compels many to deny problems, retreat into further isolation, and even resort to alcohol or other drugs for respite (Atkinson, Ganzin, & Bernstein, 1992; Jinks & Raschko, 1990). Specific risk factors of alcohol problems among older men are stressors involving finances, few resources from children, extended family members, and friends. Women problem drinkers report more negative life events, more ongoing difficulties with spouses and extended family members, and fewer resources from spouses as stressors (Atkinson, 1994; Brennan & Moos, 1990; Moos, Brennan, & Moos, 1991).

The issues associated with chronic alcohol dependency and associated health problems among older adults are poorly understood. Although the percentage of older adults with alcohol problems, when compared to current cohorts of younger adults, is not high, the actual number of older individuals with alcohol problems will increase as the demographic trends continue. Research is needed to provide a knowledge base: (a) to understand the roles of gender, ethnic group membership, psychosocial, and socioeconomic factors in the development of alcohol problems, and (b) to inform the political debates that determine health policy for older adults.

Rehabilitation Issues

The goal in caring for older adults is fundamentally rehabilitative (Williams, 1990). It has long been known that physical exercise and mental activity can restore functions lost through inactivity. Rehabilitation for older adults must maximize the autonomy of the individual, be based on life history and personality development, develop collaborative partnerships, and be designed to accommodate the continued support required by chronic conditions. Older adults with debilitating disorders confront the societal attitudes about aging and disability. There are powerful myths and stereotypes about aging that limit the management of chronic illnesses in older adults and limit the perceived value of rehabilitation for this population. Age is viewed as something to be postponed, denied, and devalued. Ageism teaches that to be old is to be ill and incurable (Alford & Futrell, 1992). Research with older adults contradicts this idea. Many older adults report being "healthy" or "very healthy," and base this belief on their ability to function not only at a basic level required for everyday living, but also to engage in sports and to travel (Catanzaro, 1990). The "biomedicalization of aging" (Binney, Estes, & Ingman, 1990; Estes & Binney, 1989) has propelled health care for older adults into care that creates dependency rather than self-care and independence. In the 1992 Kent Lecture, Estes (1993) outlined a framework for empowering older adults and negating the negative effects of the biomedicalization of aging. A key component of this framework is rehabilitation and the restoration of independent functioning of older adults through carefully designed and tested interventions, such as those for stroke, hip fracture, and urinary incontinence (Estes, 1993; Ory & Williams, 1989).

Becker and Kaufman (1988, p. 459) suggest that rehabilitation services are not offered to older adults because "the restoration of normal function and return to self-sufficiency is thought to be unlikely among elderly persons. Moreover, the failures of elderly persons to return to former levels of function is considered acceptable and even appropriate in American society." There is evidence to suggest that the level of preillness or preaccident functioning affects the type of rehabilitation (Brody & Ruff, 1986), and the level of cognitive impairment influences decisions to provide rehabilitative services, that is, diminished cognitive ability translates into less rehabilitation (Schuman, Beattie, Steed, Merry, & Kraus, 1981). Current standard rehabilitation goals often limit access of older adults to rehabilitative services. When outcomes of rehabilitation are oriented toward full-time employment, older retired adults are by definition excluded from these services (Myers, 1985, 1994).

The research base on aging, chronic illness, and rehabilitation outcomes is very limited. Nevertheless, there are data, albeit sketchy, that provide evidence that four factors affect the accessibility to and outcomes of rehabilitation services for older adults with chronic illnesses. These are (1) age, (2) gender, (3) public policy (principally health care reimbursement), and (4) professional priorities.

Age

Age per se has failed to predict the sequelae of major disabilities or the outcomes of rehabilitation. Nevertheless, it has been used as a reason for excluding older adults from rehabilitative services. A study of 708 people with spinal cord injury, ranging in age from 6 to 88, demonstrated no effect of age and skill performance for those with complete or incomplete quadriplegia or incomplete paraplegia. For those with complete paraplegia, there was an age-associated decrease in independence in bathing, dressing, stair climbing, and transferring to chair, toilet, and bath (Yarkony, Roth, Heinemann, & Lovell, 1988). Twenty-two of 26 older persons with significant closed head injury were discharged from a rehabilitation program to their homes, and more than half of them were independent in activities of daily living (Davis & Acton, 1988). The rehabilitation experience of an inpatient stroke rehabilitation program demonstrated that adults aged 65 to 75 were admitted to rehabilitation earlier, and with comparable cognitive but poorer motor function, than were adults under age 65. Rehabilitation intensity and type were similar across age groups. However, older adults had significantly shorter rehabilitation stays and had poorer motor function at discharge, which may have contributed to the older group more often being discharged to a nursing home or requiring a paid caregiver. The authors concluded that the effect of frailty and comorbid disease upon stroke disability may explain the findings (Falconer, Naughton, Strasser, & Sinacore, 1994). These findings may also be attributed to a pervasive belief that older adults cannot benefit or do not benefit from rehabilitation services and thus were provided less service than their younger counterparts. Left unanswered by the study was whether, given the same length of a rehabilitation program, the older group would have come closer to the achievements of the younger group.

Research in the area of aging and rehabilitation has lagged far behind research in other areas of aging, in spite of the knowledge that excess functional disability of chronic health problems can be diminished with appropriate rehabilitation. Critical questions remain unanswered about the role of physical and mental conditioning in preventing, slowing, or reversing age-related changes in function (Institute of Medicine, 1991). Knowledge of the outcomes of rehabilitation for subgroups of older adults, such as women and people of color, is virtually unknown because of the absence of research in geriatric rehabilitation. The cost-effectiveness of delivering rehabilitation care in institutions versus the community has not been addressed adequately.

The majority of rehabilitation research has focused on outcomes, such as full-time employment, that are inappropriate for older adults. Significant work has been done on older adults who have suffered a stroke. Far less attention has been paid to older adults who suffered a stroke as young or middle-aged adults, or older adults who acquired a disability in youth or middle age as a result of trauma, such as spinal cord and brain injuries, and must now incorporate their residual disability with aging changes.

Gender

Gender makes a difference in how a person is perceived and what choices are possible (Hess, 1990). Women 75 years of age and older are more likely than men to have a disability. Under age 70, men are more likely than women to be limited in major activity (LaPlante, 1992). Gender has not been shown to influence independence in activities of daily living. Women, however, particularly older women, are disadvantaged in their access to rehabilitation resources (Ades, Waldmann, Polk, & Coflesky, 1992; Altman & Smith, 1990, 1992). For example, Altman and Smith demonstrated that uneducated white women, regardless of age, have less access to rehabilitation resources. And as noted earlier, older women are less likely to be referred to cardiac rehabilitation programs than men with similar disease severity (Young & Kahana, 1993).

Public Policy Factors

Several public policy factors further compromise the ability of older adults to obtain rehabilitative services. Lack of reimbursement at the federal and state levels for rehabilitative services jeopardizes the ability of health care professionals to assist older adults to maximize their independence in the least restrictive environment. There is little realization that rehabilitation of older adults is consistent with the public policy objective of conserving resources (Betts, 1990).

Professional Priorities

Priorities established by health care professions favor the use of advanced technology over time-honored rehabilitation strategies (Joseph & Wanlass, 1993). Many primary care providers for older adults lack knowledge of the principles of geriatric rehabilitation (Hoenig, 1993; Rodriguez & Goldberg,

1993). In general, health sciences curricula fall short of equipping graduates to understand either geriatrics or rehabilitation and little is done to integrate the two fields of study (Hoenig).

In summary, as the population ages the prevalence of chronic diseases and their disabling sequelae will continue to escalate. Research has shown that age alone is not predictive of either disability or rehabilitation outcomes. The persistence of myths and stereotypes about age and disability, and the continuing emphasis in health professional schools on high-technology care, will continue to compromise quality of life for older adults with disabilities resulting from chronic illness. Health care policies at the state and federal levels erect significant barriers to the delivery of appropriate rehabilitative services to older adults. Without significant changes in public policy, research dollars will continue to be directed toward medical conditions that can result in mortality, rather than those with morbidity and disability outcomes that could be ameliorated by rehabilitation services.

PUBLIC POLICY, AGING, AND CHRONIC ILLNESS: FUTURE DIRECTIONS

The present system of health care does not promote quality care for older adults with chronic health problems. Significant changes in public policy are needed to ensure the equitable and just distribution of health services to older adults as we move into the 21st century. Major areas of concern have been reviewed in this chapter. They can be summarized in three categories, each with significant, if not profound, implications for current and future health care for older adults:

1. demographic trends toward an increasingly older population;
2. the current social, political, and economic context of health care, which accounts for the biases in health care for women, the poor, and people of color; and
3. the impact of the current health care context on the delivery of mental health care and rehabilitation for older adults.

Two recurring themes in these discussions are the current emphasis on acute illness care accompanied by a deemphasis on chronic conditions, and the high cost of and poor access to health care.

These factors are highly interrelated, and one cannot be discussed in isolation from the others. Nor can policy changes be made to address any one of these factors without considering all. Given this "web of causation" (Estes & Rundall, 1992), it is difficult to propose specific policy changes that will address each concern. Overall, profound changes in the prevailing, underlying, philosophical beliefs and assumptions about old age and morbidity/mortality, acute/chronic, cure/care, "high tech"/"high touch," and accommodation/rehabilitation will be essential to revise the current directions in health care for older adults with chronic illnesses.

Estes (1993) and Estes, Swan, and Associates (1993) describe the new directions for social policy and community care for older adults as the "empowerment imperative." Although this term is used in reference to social policy, it is applicable as well to the philosophical and practical changes necessary for future health care for older adults. The empowerment imperative is defined as "a commitment to the design and evaluation of social *and health* interventions that enhance the capacity of the old and chronically ill for self-esteem, personal control, individual and social involvement. . . . The commitment is also to the development of interventions that modify the structural conditions (e.g., health policy) that contribute to or generate dependency in old age" (Estes, p. 294, emphasis added).

The belief that aging and disease are synonymous, and that decline is inevitable, must change. This belief drives the current focus on acute, highly technical, and costly medical care at curing disease. The success of current health care in decreasing mortality or increasing longevity should be acknowledged, but at the same time this question must be raised: Have these successes contributed to extended years of quality life, or to extended years of disability (Verbrugge, 1984)? New directions for health care for older adults must be based on the conviction that extension of life is not the only goal, or even the highest goal of quality health care. Future care must focus on programs and policies that increase elders' choices and self-care and decrease dependence on medical/health caregivers. This means that policies are needed that direct program and research funding toward community-based care and the social and health services that promote and ensure maximum years of independent living (Estes, 1993). In this approach to health care, the emphasis would be on rehabilitation for maximum function, rather than on accommodating to disability, a subtle but important distinction.

Major rethinking, redirection, and revisions of health and social policies that currently discriminate against women, the poor, and people of color will be needed to ensure that the social, political, and economic structures work to the benefit of all citizens. Access to care for all older adults can only be assured when costs of care are controlled and opportunities for quality care do not depend on gender, race, or financial status. The current two-tiered system of health care—one for those who can pay the rising costs and one for those who are poor or near poor, for whom there are increasingly limited care options—must be eliminated. Equitable access to mental health care must be assured, and health practitioners must be trained adequately to recognize and treat appropriately mental health problems in older adults. Exploitation of caregiving women, whose work enables the nation to avoid formally paying the cost of long-term care, must end and "gender justice" must begin (Estes & Rundall, 1992). So-called color-blind care (Yee, 1992) must be replaced by culturally sensitive care, where individual belief systems and values are an integral component of the care.

In sum, population aging has major implications for changes in the health care needs of the future. Failure to plan for these changes will result in costly and inequitable distribution of health services for this population. Significant new directions in health care for older adults cannot be achieved without significant changes in social, political, and economic policies and structures that determine the delivery of health care. Nurses, as the major health care professionals providing care to older adults, are in a position to influence the future direction of their health care. How we make our influence felt will depend on our commitment to this population, our knowledge of its health needs, our willingness to become politically involved, and the sophistication of our participation in the political process.

REFERENCES

Abraham, I., Buckwalter, K., Neese, J., & Fox, J. (1994). Mental health of rural elderly: A research agenda for nursing. *Issues in Mental Health Nursing, 15*(3), 203–213.

Adams, W. L., Magruder-Habib, K., Trued, S., & Broome, H. (1992). Alcohol abuse in elderly emergency department patients. *Journal of the American Geriatrics Society, 40,* 1236–1240.

Adams, W. L., Yuan, Z., Barboriak, J. J., & Rimm, A. A. (1993). Alcohol related hospitalizations of elderly people. *Journal of the American Medical Association, 270(*10), 6–9.

Ades, P. A., Waldmann, M. L., Polk, D. M., & Coflesky, J. T. (1992). Referral patterns and exercise response in the rehabilitation of female coronary patients aged greater than or equal to 62 years. *American Journal of Cardiology, 69,* 1422–1425.

Alford, D. M., & Futrell, M. (1992). Wellness and health promotion of the elderly. *Nursing Outlook, 40,* 221–226.

Altman, B. M., & Smith, R. T. (1990). Rehabilitation service utilization models: Changes in the opportunity structure for disabled women. *International Journal of Rehabilitation Research, 12,* 149–156.

Altman, B. M., & Smith, R. T. (1992). Impact of rehabilitation on psychological distress: Gender differences. *International Journal of Rehabilitation Research, 15,* 75–81.

American Psychiatric Association. (1994). *Diagnostic and statistical manual of mental disorders* (4th ed.). Washington, DC: Author.

Anthony, J., & Aboraya, A. (1992). The epidemiology of selected mental disorders in later life. In J. Birren, R. Sloane, & G. Cohen (Eds.), *Handbook of mental health and aging* (2nd ed., pp. 27–73). San Diego, CA: Academic Press.

Arendell, T., & Estes, C. (1991). Older women in the post-Reagan era. *International Journal of Health Services, 21*(1), 59–73.

Atkinson, R. M. (1990). Aging and alcohol use disorders: Diagnostic issues in the elderly. *International Psychogeriatrics, 2*(1), 55–72.

Atkinson, R. M. (1994). Late onset problem drinking in older adults. *International Journal of Geriatric Psychiatry, 9*(4), 321–326.

Atkinson, R. M., Ganzini, L., & Bernstein, M. (1992). Alcohol and substance use disorders in the elderly. In J. Birren, R. Sloane, & G. Cohen (Eds.), *Handbook of mental health and aging* (2nd ed., pp. 515–555). San Diego, CA: Academic Press.

Ayanian, J., & Epstein, A. (1991). Differences in the use of procedures between women and men hospitalized for coronary heart disease. *New England Journal of Medicine, 325,* 221–225.

Becker, G., & Kaufman, S. (1988). Old age, rehabilitation, and research: A review of the issues. *Gerontologist, 28*(4), 459–468.

Betts, H. B. (1990). Rehabilitation and the elderly: A psychiatrist's view. In S. J. Brody & G. E. Ruff (Eds.), *Aging and rehabilitation: Advances in the state of the art* (pp. 30–43). New York: Springer.

Binney, E., Estes, C., & Ingman, S. (1990). Medicalization, public policy and the elderly: Social services in jeopardy? *Social Science and Medicine, 30*(7), 761–771.

Blazer, D., Hughes, D., & George, L. (1987). The epidemiology of depression in an elderly community population. *Gerontologist, 27* (2), 281–287.

Blume, S. (1990). Chemical dependency in women: Important issues. *American Journal of Drug and Alcohol Abuse, 16,* 297–303.

Booth, B., Blow, F., Cook, C., Bunn, J., & Fortney, J. (1992). Age and ethnicity among hospitalized alcoholics: A nationwide study. *Alcoholism: Clinical and Experimental Research, 16*(6), 1029–1034.

Brennan, P. L., & Moos, R. H. (1990). Life stressors, social resources, and late-life problem drinking. *Psychology in Aging, 5*(4), 491–501.

Brennan, P. L., Moos, R. H., & Kim, Y. J. (1993). Gender differences in the individual characteristics and life contexts of late-middle-aged and older problem drinkers. *Addiction, 88,* 781–790.

Brody, S. J., & Ruff, G. E. (Eds.). (1986). *Aging and rehabilitation: Advances in the state of the art.* New York: Springer.

Burkhauser, R. (1994). Protecting the most vulnerable: A proposal to improve Social Security insurance for older women. *Gerontologist, 34*(2), 148–149.

Burns, C. M. (1994). Early detection and intervention for the hidden alcoholic: Assessment guidelines for the clinical nurse specialist. *Journal for Advanced Nursing Practice, 8*(6), 296–303.

Caetano, R. (1989). Drinking patterns and alcohol problems in a national sample of U.S. Hispanics. In D. Spiegler, D. Tate, S. Aitken, & C. Christian (Eds.), *Alcohol use among U.S. minorities* (NIAAA Research Monograph No. 18. DHHS Publication No. ADM 89–1435). Washington, DC: U.S. Government Printing Office.

Callahan, C., Hui, S., Nienaber, N., Musick, B., & Tierney, W. (1994). Longitudinal study of depression and health services use among elderly primary care patients. *Journal of the American Geriatrics Society, 42*(8), 833–838.

Casey, D. (1994). Depression in the elderly. *Southern Medical Journal, 87*(5), 559–563.

Catanzaro, M. (1990, May). *What does it mean to be healthy? The perspective of leisure participants.* Paper presented at the Communicating Nursing Research Conference, Denver, CO.

Cloninger, C., Bohman, M., & Sigvardsson, S. (1981). Inheritance of alcohol abuse. *Archives of General Psychiatry, 38,* 861–868.

Cloninger, C., Reich, T., Sigvardsson, S., Von Knoring, A., & Bohman, M. (1987). The effects of changes in alcohol use between generations on the inheritance of alcohol abuse. In R. Ross & J. Barrett (Eds.), *Alcoholism: Origins and outcomes* (pp. 49–74). New York: Raven Press.

Commonwealth Fund Survey of Women's Health. (1993). New York: Commonwealth Fund.

Conwell, Y., Rotenberg, M., & Caine, E. (1990). Completed suicide at age 50 and over. *Journal of the American Geriatrics Society, 38*(6), 640–644.

Davis, C. S., & Acton, P. (1988). Treatment of elderly brain-injured patients. Experience in a traumatic brain injury unit. *Journal of the American Geriatric Society, 36,* 225–229.

Dimond, M. (1995). Older women's health. In C. Fogel & N. F. Woods (Eds.), *Women's health care* (pp. 101–110). Thousand Oaks, CA: Sage.

Dimond, M., Caserta, M., & Lund, D. (1994). Understanding depression in bereaved older adults. *Clinical Nursing Research, 3*(3), 253–268.

Dufour, M., Archer, L., & Gordis, E. (1992). Alcohol and the elderly. *Clinics in Geriatric Medicine, 8*(1), 127–141.

Estes, C. (1993). The aging enterprise revisited. *Gerontologist, 33*(3), 292–298.

Estes, C., & Binney, E. (1989). The biomedicalization of aging: Dangers and dilemmas. *Gerontologist, 29,* 587–596.

Estes, C., & Rundall, T. (1992). Social characteristics, social structures, and health in the aging population. In M. Ory, R. Abeles, & P. Lipman (Eds.), *Aging, health and behavior* (pp. 299–326). Newbury Park, CA: Sage.

Estes, C., Swan, R., & Associates (Eds.). (1993). *The long term care crisis*. Newbury Park, CA: Sage.

Falconer, J. A., Naughton, B. J., Strasser, D. C., & Sinacore, J. M. (1994). Stroke inpatient rehabilitation: A comparison across age groups. *Journal of the American Geriatrics Society, 42*(1), 39–44.

Frank-Stromberg, M. (1991). Changing demographics in the United States: Implications for health professionals. *Cancer, 67*(Suppl. 6), 1772–1778.

Gelfand, D., & Baressi, C. (1987). Current perspectives in ethnicity and aging. In D. Gelfand & C. Baressi (Eds.), *Ethnic dimensions of aging* (pp. 5–17). New York: Springer.

Gilford, D. (Ed.). (1988). *The aging population in the twenty-first century*. Washington, DC: National Academy Press.

Goldberg, E., Van Natta, P., & Comstock, G. (1985). Depressive symptoms, social networks, and social support of elderly women. *American Journal of Epidemiology, 121*(3), 448–456.

Gurland, E., Dean, L., Cross, P., & Golden, R. (1980). The epidemiology of depression and dementia in the elderly: The use of multiple indicators. In J. Cole & J. Barrett (Eds.), *Psychopathology in the aged* (pp. 37–62). New York: Raven Press.

Hafner, H., & Weyerer, S. (1986). Mental health in the aged [(English abstract)]. *Wiener, Klinische, Wochenschrift, 98*(19), 635–642.

Heath, D. B. (1989). American Indians and alcohol: Epidemiological and sociocultural relevance. In D. L. Spiegler, D. A. Tate, S. S. Aitken, & C. M. Christian (Eds.), *Alcohol use among U.S. Minorities* (NIAAA Research Monograph No. 18. DHHS Publication No. ADM 89–1435). Washington, DC: U.S. Government Printing Office.

Herd, D. (1990). Subgroup differences in drinking patterns among black and white men: Results from a national survey. *Journal of Studies in Alcohol, 51,* 221–232.

Hess, B. B. (1990). Preface. In E. R. Rosenthal (Ed.), *Women aging and ageism* (pp. xi–xiii). Binghamton, NY: Haworth Press.

Heston, L., Garrard, J., Makris, L., Kane, R., Cooper, S., Dunham, T., & Zelterman, D. (1992). Inadequate treatment of depressed nursing home elderly. *Journal of the American Geriatrics Society, 40*(11), 1117–1122.

Hill, R., Gallagher, D., Thompson, L., & Ishida, T. (1988). Hopelessness as a measure of suicidal intent in the depressed elderly. *Psychology and Aging, 3*(3), 230–232.

Hisnanick, J., & Erickson, P. (1993). Hospital resource utilization by American Indians/Alaska Natives for alcoholism and alcohol abuse. *American Journal of Drug and Alcohol Abuse, 19*(3), 387–396.

Hoenig, H. (1993). Educating primary care physicians in geriatric rehabilitation. *Clinical Geriatric Medicine, 9*(4), 883–893.

Holzer, C. E., III, Robins, L., Myers, J., Weissman, M., Tischler, G., Leaf, P., Anthony, J., & Bednarski, P. (1984). Antecedents and correlates of alcohol abuse and dependence in the elderly. In G. Maddox, L. Robins, & N. Rosenberg, (Eds.), *Nature and extent of alcohol problems among the elderly* (pp. 217–244, Research Monograph No. 14, U.S. Department of Health and Human Services, Alcohol, Drug Abuse, and Mental Health Administration, National Institute of Alcohol Abuse and Alcoholism). Rockville, MD: U.S. Government Printing Office.

Hopper, S. (1993). The influence of ethnicity on the health of older women. *Clinical Geriatric Medicine, 9*(1), 231–259.

Institute of Medicine. (1991). *Extending life, enhancing life: A national research agenda on aging.* Washington, DC: National Academy Press.

Jinks, M. J., & Raschko, R. R. (1990) A profile of alcohol and prescription drug abuse in a high-risk community-based elderly population. *DICP, Annals of Pharmacotherapy, 24,* 971–975.

Johnson, C. (1994). Differential expectations and realities: Race, socioeconomic status and health of the oldest-old. *International Journal of Aging and Human Development, 38*(1), 13–27.

Joseph, C. L., & Wanlass, W. (1993). Rehabilitation in the nursing home. *Clinics in Geriatric Medicine, 9*(4), 859–871.

Kemp, B. J., Staples, F., & López-Aqueres, W. (1987). Epidemiology of depression and dysphoria in an elderly Hispanic population. *Journal of the American Geriatrics Society, 35,* 920–926.

Koenig, H., & Blazer, D. (1992). Epidemiology of geriatric affective disorders. *Clinics in Geriatric Medicine, 8*(2), 235–251.

LaPlante, M. P. (1992, December). *Disability Statistics Abstract,* No. 5. San Francisco: Disability Statistics Program.

Lawson, G. W., & Lawson, A. W. (1993). *Alcoholism and substance abuse in special populations.* San Diego, CA: United States International University.

Lombardo, N. (1994). *Barriers to mental health services for nursing home residents.* Washington, DC: American Association of Retired Persons.

McKenna, M. (1989). Twice in need of care: A transcultural nursing analysis of elderly Mexican Americans. *Journal of Transcultural Nursing, 1*(1), 46–52.

Miller, N. S., Belkin, B. M., & Gold, M. S. (1991). Alcohol and drug dependence among the elderly: Epidemiology, diagnosis and treatment. *Comprehensive Psychiatry, 32*(2), 153–165.

Moos, R. H., Brennan, P. L., & Moos, B. S. (1991). Short-term processes of remission and nonremission among late-life problem drinkers. *Alcoholism: Clinical Experimental Research, 15,* 948–955.

Morton, D., Schoenrock, S., Stanford, E. P., Peddecord, K., & Molgaard, C. (1989). Use of the CES-D among a community sample of older Mexican-Americans. *Journal of Cross-Cultural Gerontology, 4,* 289–306.

Muller, C. (1988). Medicaid: The lower tier of health care for women. *Women and Health, 14*(2), 81–102.

Murrell, S., Himmelfarb, S., & Wright, K. (1983). Prevalence of depression and its correlates in older adults. *American Journal of Epidemiology, 117*(2), 173–185.

Myers, J. E. (1994). Education and training of aged-care providers. *Disability Rehabilitation, 16*(3), 171–180.

Myers, J. E. (1985). Rehabilitation of older people. *Annual Review of Rehabilitation, 4,* 1–54.

National Center for Health Statistics. (1988). Advance report of final mortality statistics, 1986. *NCHS Monthly Vital Statistics Report, 37*(Suppl. 6).

National Center for Health Statistics. (1990). *Health of black and white Americans.* Atlanta: Center for Disease Control.

National Center for Health Statistics. (1986). Health statistics of older persons, United States. *Vital and health statistics* (Series 3, No. 25). Washington, DC.

Ory, M., & Williams, T. F. (1989). Rehabilitation: Small goals and sustained interventions. *Annals of the American Academy of Political and Social Sciences, 5,* 60–71.

Parmelee, P., Katz, I., & Lawton, M. P. (1989). Depression among institutionalized aged: Assessment and prevalence estimation. *Journal of Gerontology, 44*(1), M22–29.

Perales, C. (1988). Introduction. *Women and Health, 14*(2), 1–20.

Preston, S., & Martin, L. (1994). Introduction. In L. Martin & S. Preston (Eds.), *Demography of aging*. Washington, DC: National Academy Press.

Prospective Payment Assessment Commission. (1989). *Medicare prospective payment and the American health care system: Report to the Congress, June 1989.* Washington, DC: U.S. Government Printing Office.

Quinn, J. (1987). The economic status of the elderly: Beware the mean. *Review of Income and Wealth, 33,* 63–82.

Quinn, J., & Smeeding, T. (1993). The present and future of economic well-being of the aged. In R. Burkhauser & D. Salisbury (Eds.), *Pensions in a changing economy* (pp. 5–18). Washington, DC: Employee Benefits Research Institute.

Rabins, P. (1992). Prevention of mental disorder in the elderly: Current perspectives and future prospects. *Journal of the American Geriatrics Society, 40*(7), 727–737.

Radner, D. (1992). *Assessment of the economic state of the aged* (Office of Research and Statistics Working Paper No. 55). Washington, DC: Social Security Administration.

Rapp, S., & Davis, K. (1989). Geriatric depression: Physicians' knowledge, perceptions and diagnostic practices. *Gerontologist, 29*(2), 252–257.

Rice, D., Kelman, S., Miller, L., & Dunmeyer, S. (1990). *The economic costs of alcohol and drug abuse and mental illness: 1985* (DHHS Publication No. ADM 90–1694). National Institute on Alcohol Abuse and Alcoholism. Washington, DC: U.S. Government Printing Office.

Ries, D. (1987). *Health care coverage by age, sex, race and family income: U.S. 1986.* Washington, DC: National Center for Health Statistics.

Robins, L. N., Helzer, J. E., Przybeck, T. R., & Reigier, D. (1988). Alcohol disorders in the community: A report from the epidemiologic catchment area. In R. Rose & J. Barret (Eds.), *Alcoholism: Origins and outcomes* (pp. 15–29). New York: Raven Press.

Rodriguez, G. S., & Goldberg, B. (1993). Rehabilitation in the outpatient setting. *Clinical Geriatric Medicine, 9*(4), 873–881.

Schonfeld, L., & Dupree, L. (1991). Antecedents of drinking for early-and late-onset elderly alcohol abusers. *Journal of Studies on Alcohol, 52*(6), 587–592.

Schuman, J., Beattie, E., Steed, D., Merry, G., & Kraus, A. (1981). Geriatric patients with and without intellectual dysfunction: Effectiveness of a standard rehabilitation program. *Archives of Physical Medicine and Rehabilitation, 62,* 612–618.

Sofaer, S., & Abel, E. (1990). Older women's health and financial vulnerability: Implications of the Medicare benefit structure. *Women and Health, 16*(3-4), 47–66.

Stanford, E. P., & Du Bois, B. (1992). Gender and ethnicity patterns. In J. Birren, R. Sloane, & G. Cohen (Eds.), *Handbook of mental health and aging* (2nd ed., pp. 99–117). San Diego, CA: Academic Press.

Taeuber, C. (1992). Sixty-five plus in America. *Current Population Reports* (Series P–23, No. 178). Washington, DC: U.S. Government Printing Office.

Task Force on Older Women's Health. (1993). Older women's health. *Journal of the American Geriatrics Society, 41*(6), 680–683.

Tobin, J., Wasertheil-Smoller, S., Wexler, J., Steingart, R., Budner, N., Lense, L., & Wachspress, J. (1987). Sex bias when considering coronary by-pass surgery. *Annals of Internal Medicine, 107*(1), 19–25.

United Nations. (1993). *World population trends and prospects: The 1992 revision.* New York: Author.

U.S. Congress. (1991). *Aging America: Trends and projections: 1991.* Senate Special Committee on Aging. Washington, DC: U.S. Government Printing Office.

U.S. Department of Commerce. (1992). Poverty in the United States: 1991. *Current Population Reports* (Series P-60, No. 181). Washington, DC: U.S. Government Printing Office.

Verbrugge, L. (1984). Longer life but worsening health? Trends in health and mortality of middle-aged and older persons. *Milbank Memorial Fund Quarterly, 62,* 475–519.

Verbrugge, L., & Patrick, D. (1995). Seven chronic conditions: Their impact on U.S. adults' activity levels and use of medical services. *American Journal of Public Health, 85*(2), 173–182.

Weissman, M., Bruce, M., Leaf, P., Florio, L., & Holzer, C., III. (1991). Affective disorders. In L. Robins & D. Regier (Eds.), *Psychiatric disorders in America: The epidemiologic catchment area study* (pp. 53–80). New York: Free Press.

Wenger, N., Speroff, L., & Packard, B. (1993). Cardiovascular health and disease in women. *New England Journal of Medicine, 329*(4), 247–256.

Williams, T. F. (1990). Introduction to rehabilitation and aging. In S. J. Brody & L. G. Pawlson (Eds.), *Aging and rehabilitation II: The state of the practice* (pp. 3–8). New York: Springer.

Yarkony, G. M., Roth, E. J., Heinemann, A. W., & Lovell, L. L. (1988). Spinal cord injury rehabilitation outcomes: The impact of age. *Journal of Clinical Epidemiology, 41,* 173–177.

Yeatts, D., Crow, T., & Folts, E. (1992). Service use among low-income minority elderly: Strategies for overcoming barriers. *Gerontologist, 32*(1), 24–32.

Yee, D. (1992). Health care access and advocacy for immigrant and other underserved elders. *Journal of Health Care for the Poor and Underserved, 2*(4), 448–464.

Young, R., & Kahana, E. (1993). Gender, recovery from late life heart attack, and medical care. *Women and Health, 20*(1), 11–31.

CHAPTER 2

Health Promotion for Chronically Ill Elders

Joanne Sabol Stevenson*

The objective of health promotion for the chronically ill older adult is to live a full life rather than something less. Further, maintaining one's health is an ongoing process requiring a constellation of resources. Nowhere is there such an overlap among health promotion, risk reduction, and illness care as in a discussion of health promotion during chronic illness. Any such discussion is a slippery slope; a presentation about health promotion can be easily interpreted as ultimately a discussion of disease management or rehabilitation. This chapter will focus on health promoting goals and activities that are not directly focused on:

1. usual treatment of the chronic condition;
2. management of the cardinal symptoms of the condition; or
3. rehabilitation from the direct effects of that condition.

So, for example, in considering health promotion in Type II Diabetes, the diabetic diet regimen would not be considered a health promotion activity. However, nutritional guidance to enhance the intake of fruits and vegetables with more phytochemicals to fight against cancer and other diseases would be within the purview of health promotion for many chronically ill persons, including those with diabetes.

*The author wishes to acknowledge the contribution of Patricia Davis, whose able assistance in searching the literature and help with other tasks related to this review is greatly appreciated.

HEALTH PROMOTION AND CHRONIC ILLNESS: A SEEMING CONTRADICTION IN TERMS

Context and Definition

While for many, the concept of health promotion is defined narrowly as a series of activities for young populations that involve fitness programs, ideal weight attainment and maintenance, and stress management, a broader and more holistic vision of it is gaining acceptance. In 1986, at the first International Conference on Health Promotion held in Ottawa, Canada, the World Health Organization's (WHO) representatives from 14 countries of the North American and European regions developed the Ottawa Charter (Kaplun, 1992). This group of 84 representatives viewed health promotion as an enabling process, one that empowered people to increase their control over their health and to improve their total health and sense of well-being. Health, therefore, was defined as a "resource" for everyday life, not an objective to be obtained at some point in time. According to the Ottawa Charter, good health is viewed as a "resource" that goes hand in hand with social, economic, and personal development, and it is a critically important resource for attaining and maintaining a high-level quality of life (Kaplun, 1992).

Health promotion, then, comprises those actions aimed at making all conditions, internal to the person and external to the person, conducive to building up this "resource" called health (Kaplun, 1992). This implies that health personnel alone cannot be responsible for health promotion. The individual, the health care provider community, and the society as a whole are involved in making health promotion a reality. Health-promotion policy at the levels of the local community, state, nation, and world involves legislative efforts, economic efforts, organizational efforts, and educational efforts. These efforts would be directed toward ensuring safer and healthier foods, better consumer products, healthier public services, and cleaner, safer, higher quality environments. The individual is responsible for advocating his or her own health promotion, making critical decisions that are health promoting, demanding goods and services that lead toward good health, and engaging in activities on a daily basis that are health promoting. The image that generally emerges from this type of discussion involves robust, vibrantly alive young adults who are free of any physical limitations or disease conditions. But could this discussion refer as well to older persons with chronic illnesses? The idea seems to be a contradiction in terms.

The "Healthy Ill Person"

According to Milz (1992), the idea of a "healthy ill person" is a perceptual challenge for the ill person, the family, the care provider, and the public. Health care personnel are accustomed to focusing on those components (body systems) of the person that are diseased or disturbed and tend to overlook that which is not ill, even though it is the greater aspect of the person. Further, within the overly specialized and fragmented health care system, all parties focus on treating the pathological condition and ignore the myriad opportunities to focus on health promotion. In dealing with people with heart disease, for example, it is very important to address breast self-examination, pelvic examination, Papanicolaou tests for women, testicular self-examinations for men, good nutrition including the five recommended servings of vegetables and fruits each day, exercise for balance and strength (in contrast to only aerobics for cardiac rehabilitation), and general socio-emotional well-being.

The "healthy elderly ill person" presents a conceptual and perceptual anomaly for many, if not most, health care providers. In the milieu of ageism, which pervades most health care systems, the very state of *being old* is antithetical to *being healthy* (Lauder, 1993) or *having the "resource" of health* (Kaplun, 1992). Age equates with disease in most providers' minds and in most chronically ill elders' minds as well. Elders themselves, like the majority of the public and most care providers, believe that many of the untoward events they experience are the natural consequences of old age, when in fact they are the results of unhealthy lifestyles or genetically predisposed conditions. Generally speaking, the aged chronically ill in today's society suffer much more than is necessary. They are more disabled than their chronic conditions warrant, and they are less functionally independent than they should be even with a chronic illness. The burden of responsibility for this situation does not lie totally on the health care community or any other single entity. However, the health care providers, as the professionally trained group, can and should take steps to intervene and ameliorate the situation with all due speed. Healthy ill persons, according to the Ottawa Charter, are people seeking a new way of life; health promotion is not a new medical treatment, but a social, ecological, and holistic concept (Milz, 1992). The challenge of health promotion for chronically ill older adults thus rests coequally on the individuals with chronic illness, their health care providers, the policy makers, and the general public.

CORRELATES OF A HEALTH-PROMOTING LIFESTYLE

What are some characteristics of elders who engage in health-promoting lifestyles? Resiliency, hardiness, concerns about events in the world, and meta-aging issues that focused on personal growth were the factors noted by elders who considered themselves to have higher levels of wellness in a south Florida study (Miller, 1991). Duffy (1993) found that the three determinants of a health-promoting lifestyle in older persons, which accounted for 89% of the variance, were (1) a positive belief about controllability of their own health, (2) higher self-esteem, and (3) internal locus of control. Unfortunately for men who had health problems, these determinants plus higher income were less likely to lead to health-promoting activities. This finding suggests that men experiencing poorer health see themselves as less able to benefit from health-promoting activities. However, there is considerable evidence to suggest that this is an inaccurate perception; indeed, the evidence suggests that health-promoting activities might go a long way toward increasing the quality of life for persons with chronic conditions (Kaplun, 1992).

For elderly persons with disabilities, the strongest predictors of engaging in a health-promoting lifestyle were higher self-efficacy for health behaviors, a wellness-oriented definition of health, less need for mechanical assistance (e.g., a walker), and being female (Stuifbergen & Becker, 1994). The disabled males were less likely than their disabled female counterparts to embrace a health-promoting lifestyle. Older men also seemed to put less value on health (Whetstone & Reid, 1991) than their female counterparts. Older African American women, however, decreased their health-promoting activities once they began to become functionally disabled (Ferraro, 1993). So there is considerable evidence that the attitude of the elders is a more powerful influence than the nature or severity of the illness or disability. This finding provides a challenge to health care providers to help elders develop trust that engaging in health-promoting lifestyles will decelerate the disabling aspects of their chronic conditions.

A number of investigators have used Pender's (1982) model of health promotion as the basis for building predictive models of the tendency to engage in health-promoting activities (Duffy, 1993; Foster, 1992; Stuifbergen & Becker, 1994). Often these investigators used the Health-Promoting Lifestyle Profile (Walker, Sechrist, & Pender, 1987) as their instrument. In most studies there was a strong positive relationship between perception of current health and engaging in a health-promoting lifestyle (Duffy, 1993; Kotthoff-Burrell, 1992; Miller, 1991; Stuifbergen & Becker, 1994). An exception to this general finding from majority populations occurred among African American women. Foster found that positive perception of health did not correlate with health-promoting behaviors among an elderly sample of African American women. Further, in a study of 3,237 African American elders, Ferraro (1993) found that the African American women were exceptionally health pessimistic, had higher medical needs, and engaged less than predicted in health-promoting activities. Thus there may be culturally based challenges facing health providers when working with chronically ill elderly minorities, especially African American women. The investigators postulated that past difficulties with access to care and less belief in the United States' health care system may underlie the greater health pessimism in this population. But it could also have a deeper cultural history and be related to negative expectations about feeling good in old age.

HEALTH PROFESSIONALS AS HEALTH PROMOTION FACILITATORS

Unfortunately, there is evidence that health care professionals do not optimize the opportunities accorded to them to do health-promotion teaching, facilitation, or reinforcement while they are interacting with chronically ill elders. Surveys of primary care physicians (Black & Kapoor, 1990; Radecki & Mendenhall, 1986; Wechsler, Levine, Idelson, Rohman, & Taylor, 1983) showed extremely low rates of health-promotion counseling during office visits by chronically ill older adults.

Russell and Roter (1993) analyzed 439 audiotapes of office visits from 11 states; the patients were more often female, 59% were African American, and the most common conditions were hypertension, coronary disease, diabetes mellitus, and chronic obstructive pulmonary disease (COPD). While 53% of the audiotapes contained some mention of a health-promoting action, the overwhelming majority of these were about diet or weight control directly tied to the primary disease. Other topics received significantly less attention: 21% mentioned physical activity, 18% spoke of stress, only 12% discussed smoking cessation, and a mere 6% dealt with alcohol consumption. Most of the discussions centered around the specific disease rather than global health promotion; for example, providers discussed diet in the context of the diabetic diet or smoking in the context of COPD. None of the providers used strategies lauded in the literature to facilitate major lifestyle change—strategies such as goal setting and patient contracting. Rather, the strategy used most often was providing a verbal rationale for the lifestyle change, sometimes followed by instructions for successfully implementing the change. Compared to physicians, nurse practitioners are thought to use a wider repertoire of strategies to evoke major lifestyle changes among their clients. However, they, too, apparently focus on the disease-related symptom management more often than a holistic approach to health promotion for chronically ill older adults (Russell & Roter, 1993).

In addition to primary care offices, chronically ill older adults interact with health care providers in home care, acute care hospitals, retirement villages, assisted living facilities, and nursing homes. In each of these settings, opportunities abound for staff to teach, encourage, model, and facilitate chronically ill older adults to engage in health-promoting lifestyles.

The UCLA home-care geriatric assessment and health-promotion clinical trial is a longitudinal effort seeking to clarify some contradictory outcomes from several international studies (Hall, De Beck, Johnson, & Mackinnon, 1992; McEwan, Davison, Forster, Pearson, & Stirling, 1990; Stuck, Mayer-Oakes, & Rubenstein, 1993) that showed profound improvements in life expectancy, morale, and quality of life but inconsistent findings about subsequent hospital and nursing home admissions. In the UCLA study (Rubenstein et al., 1994), geriatric nurse practitioners are working with the 215 randomized experimental group participants who were 75 years or older at intake and will be visited over 36 months at a cost of only $484 per client per year. The domains covered are physical health, functioning, oral health, quality of life, depression, coping, social network, social support, environmental safety, personal safety, and health resources utilization. This project is one to watch, for the data could be valuable as a guide to health policy decisions into the next century.

Health-promotion studies and intervention trials among nursing home residents are less common than in other settings, according to reviews of studies by Robertson (1991) and Richardson (1992). While the well-known goals of nursing home care put forth by Kane, Ouslander, and Abrass (1994) include three that speak directly to health promotion—maintaining functional independence, maximizing quality of life, and preventing acute and iatrogenic illness—the research is sparse on health promotion in the nursing home setting. Those investigators who implemented exercise interventions with nursing home residents found positive results (Fiatarone et al., 1990; Jirovec, 1991; McMurdo & Rennie, 1993). Generally, the exercise series must start mildly and continue over many months to show measurable improvements, but patience and persistence produce remarkable outcomes (Stevenson, 1988).

The dearth of nursing home research on health promotion may be due to a timing problem. Researchers and research utilization on the basic care problems of nursing home residents have been addressed only for the past 15 years as part of the teaching nursing home concept. It may be too early for that group of investigators to turn their energies away from care research and toward health-promotion research.

It is time for long-term care researchers and health-promotion researchers to find each other. Collaborative studies, which focus on outcomes of health-promoting interventions in long-term care settings, would make a valuable contribution to the field. Currently, nursing home personnel have little freedom and even less incentive to innovate; they are bound by rigid federal and state policies and rules. Further, the minimal levels of staffing and low levels of educational preparation of long-term care nursing personnel make innovation highly unlikely. Indeed, the reason that long-term care is currently so rules-driven emanated from its history of being operated by undereducated or undertrained personnel. Hence it is important that well-planned and rigorously executed studies be done and the findings publicized to policy makers. The long-term care industry is more highly regulated than any other health care system, and essentially all innovations come into long-term care through governmental regulations. Thus mandating health-promoting interventions through the regulatory process is (unfortunately) the most effective way to change the long-term care system at the present time. The negative side of this suggestion is that innovation through governmental regulation usually disregards individual differences; all persons are mandated to receive the service even if it is not appropriate or needs to be given in a modified fashion. But flexibility and on-the-spot modification require judgment and decision making by well-trained professional staff, and that is not the reality of the long-term care system today.

REDUCTION OF FRAILTY: THE INTERMEDIARY TO DISABILITY

Buchner and Wagner (1992) defined frailty as a state of reduced physiological reserve predictive of increased susceptibility to disability. It is a state of vulnerability, fragility, and lack of resilience that precedes actual disability. In their conceptual model, chronic conditions or diseases and sedentarism (disuse syndrome) combine to lead to frailty, which in turn leads to disability.

In a large epidemiological study, Verbrugge, Lepkowski, and Imanaka (1989) found that cerebrovascular disease had the greatest impact on independent functioning of 16 conditions tested, which included cancer, fractures, and cardiac disease. Buchner and Wagner (1992) maintained that disuse syndrome (from physical inactivity) is the major accelerant of frailty and subsequent disability in the presence of chronic conditions. They cited nearly 100 studies that showed decreased or increased rate of decline depending on the level of physical and mental activity of the subjects. They denounced continued adherence to the *Rest Dogma*—the conventional wisdom that rest is the treatment for all ills—as a cardinal obstacle to preventing frailty and disability in elders (Buchner & Wagner). The contrary principle to the *Rest Dogma* is graduated, systematic, physical activity, strength training, balance and gait training, intellectual stimulation, memory training, and meaningful social interactions. They concluded that frailty, as the intermediary between chronic conditions and actual disability, can be prevented or at least delayed through interventions that target three cardinal areas: (1) neurologic and cognitive control, (2) mechanical performance, and (3) energy metabolism.

SPECIFIC TARGETS FOR HEALTH PROMOTION

Neurologic and Cognitive Control

It is believed that engaging in activities that require mental functioning, strategizing, remembering, verbal acuity, and new learning will help most people retain their cognitive and memory capacities well into very old age. In the retired population, it is essential that elders continue to make their brain cells work. Mental activities such as bridge, chess, crossword puzzles, belonging to book clubs and investment clubs, Bible study, and social interaction with a variety of people of all ages are activities that exercise cognitive processes and memory (Berry, 1994); "use it or lose it" is the principle that all older adults must live by.

Effect of Aerobic Exercise on Cognition

There are conflicting findings and an ongoing controversy about the effect of aerobic fitness training on cognitive functioning. A number of investigators have found significant improvements in several areas of cognition and short-term memory following exercise interventions (Dustman et al., 1984; Lindenmuth & Moose, 1990; Molloy, Beerschoten, et al., 1988; Stevenson & Topp, 1990; Topp & Stevenson, 1994). However, others have found no improvement (Molloy, Richardson, & Crilly, 1988; Perri & Templer, 1985). Hypotheses about why aerobic exercise would improve cognitive functioning include increased cerebral metabolic functioning, reversal of cognitive disuse syndrome, and improved integration of cerebral functioning. The problems inherent in the studies to date include testing acute effects of exercise on cognition and memory versus data collection of delayed aftereffects and mismatch of some neuropsychological test domains with the likely effects of exercise. Clearly, more finely tuned measurement and more rigorously controlled studies are needed in this area. This need becomes acute as the numbers of older adults with cognitive deficits increase and interest grows in finding viable interventions to improve or prolong cognitive abilities.

In persons with cognitive disturbances, there are myriad types and levels of disturbance and these change over time for each person. Roberts and colleagues (Roberts & Algase, 1988; Roberts & Lincoln, 1988) developed an empirically derived model of the relationship among variables related to cognitive disturbance of acute care elders and long-term care elders. The major targets for nursing intervention emanating from the model are types and foci of interactions between staff and patients and manipulation of the environment to optimize the remaining cognitive and memory capacities of the patients. The guiding principle of cognitive health promotion is intellectual and memory stimulation, with a personally meaningful purpose for each elder. It is degrading and counterproductive to coerce older adults into cognitive or memory exercises that have no utility or meaning for them (Mace, 1987). On the other hand, several investigators have shown that it is possible to maintain good cognitive function or at least decelerate losses through the application of sound cognitive interventions (Blumenthal et al., 1989; Diesfeldt & Diesfeldt-Groenendijk, 1977; Perri & Templer, 1985; Stevenson & Topp, 1990).

Alternative Therapies

An important category of health-promoting interventions is that cluster of self-care and provider-initiated activities aimed at improving one's general sense of well-being and decreasing stress and other unpleasant reactions and emotions of living with a chronic illness through the avenue of self-empowerment. A useful concept for this discussion is cognitive control, defined as mentally framing the personal situation so that it is positive and acceptable to the self (Bonnel, 1993). It differs from perceived control in that the person can have a realistic and objective view of negative states, but choose to reframe the negative as a positive. Progressive relaxation using guided imagery is proposed as a strategy that can be taught and that older persons then can use to acquire and maintain cognitive control of a variety of life situations, including symptoms, discomforts, frustrations, and hassles of their chronic illnesses.

While few controlled studies have been done, interesting preliminary findings have emerged from case (Collison & Miller, 1987), qualitative (Howell, 1994), and quasi-experimental (Slivinske & Fitch, 1987) work with elderly groups. Moody, Fraser, and Yarandi (1993) used guided imagery progressive relaxation and found improved quality of life among a group of young-old (age 55 to 64) and middle-old (age 65 to 84) adults with chronic bronchitis and emphysema. Renfroe (1988), in a randomized control study, found significant decreases in dyspnea, anxiety, heart rate, and respirations among COPD patients after 4 weeks of progressive relaxation training. Finally, other investigators (Hahn et al., 1993; Lesko & Summerfield, 1988) found that progressive relaxation and biofeedback enhanced relaxation and resulted in decreased blood pressure in borderline hypertensives.

Music is closely allied to relaxation and imagery as a therapeutic modality to promote cognitive control and improve the quality of life for older adults with chronic illnesses. In a 14-week program of relaxation, music, and art, Rosling and Kitchen (1992) found that depressed, withdrawn, and highly anxious nursing home residents responded very positively to the program and became engaged in the music and art experiences. Schorr's (1993) sample of 30 women with chronic pain from rheumatoid arthritis contained 14 older adults. These subjects reported dramatic shifts in perception of pain that occurred between the premusic and postmusic periods. There was also an enduring effect that lasted for about 2 hours postintervention.

Mechanical Performance

Strength Training, Flexibility, and Bone Density

Integrity of the musculoskeletal system is a prerequisite to normal motor functioning of the human body, which requires flexible joints, adequate muscle strength, and adequate bone strength. A synthesis of findings (Buchner & Wagner, 1992) confirmed that 25% of the variance in disability over several studies was explained by overall physical functioning status. Even hypokinetic older subjects can significantly increase their muscular strength (Fisher, Pendergast, & Calkins, 1991), balance (Sauvage et al., 1992), joint flexibility, bone density, and functional capacity (Fisher, Kame, Rouse, & Pendergast, 1994) through progressive training over 20 weeks or more (Agre, Pierce, Raab, McAdams, & Smith, 1988; Fiatarone et al., 1990, 1994; Morey, Crowley, Robbins, Cowper, & Sullivan, 1994; Nelson et al., 1994).

Perhaps due to the length of sedentarism in many frail older adults, they do not show significant progress in 4 to 6 weeks, but require 16 to 20 weeks or even more to show significant progress (Valentine-Garzon, Maynard, & Selznick, 1992). The emergent hypothesis is that the rate of adaptation of skeletal muscle to the strength training stimulus is retarded in older adults, but with patience and persistence, positive results will be forthcoming (Stamford, 1988) even in very sedentary older adults. The trick is to keep them engaged in the physical activity until results are visible to them. Measurable positive results then may become a positive reinforcer that maintains their commitment to the activity.

Energy Metabolism

Aerobic Fitness

Cardiac and pulmonary diseases are highly correlated with disability probably because they limit energy metabolism and cause fatigue and further disuse of skeletal muscles in a vicious cycle. A broad range of studies have found that maximal aerobic power is reduced in these conditions and persons cannot perform tasks that require more energy than they can produce (Buchner & Wagner, 1992). One impediment to exercise for some chronically ill groups is that they cannot exercise strenuously enough to gain the usual measurable benefits; persons with severe COPD are a case in point. A Maryland sample (Gift & Austin, 1992) and an Illinois sample of COPD patients showed improvement in functional mobility, but not because of true fitness since their level of work remained low (Kim et al., 1993). Apparently, they became less fearful and learned to tolerate more dyspnea. On the other hand, evidence exists that the cycle of low energy, further disuse, and even lower energy can be prevented or reversed in conditions such as cancer (MacVicar, Winningham, & Nickel, 1989).

Physical fitness was correlated with lower risk for all-cause and cause-specific mortality even when the subjects engaged in other nonhealthy behaviors such as smoking or had parental history of coronary heart disease (Blair et al., 1989). The effects of aerobic exercise on mild hypertension is mixed; Blumenthal, Siegel, and Appelbaum (1991) failed to find positive changes. However, their study has been criticized since only about 67% of their subjects stayed in their assigned heart rate range and many subjects had poor attendance records. So the exercise protocol in their study was probably underdosed and the findings may not be valid. Other studies of mild hypertensives showed modest gains (Alderman, 1994; Barnard, Ugianskis, & Martin, 1992).

Results of aerobic training in various cardiac populations have been more positive. Highly positive results were shown in patients with coronary artery disease by some investigators (Miller & Paffenbarger, 1992; O'Connor et al., 1989) but not others (Fletcher & Vassallo, 1993). Other groups with significant positive results included patients after cardiac transplant surgery (Kavanagh, 1992), patients following coronary artery bypass grafting or angioplasty (Foster & Tamboli, 1992), persons with angina or silent ischemia (Balady, 1992), and even patients with chronic heart failure (Adamopoulos et al., 1993; Smith, 1992).

Other investigators have shown significant positive gains from aerobic exercise for patients with Type II diabetes (Barnard et al., 1992; Leon, 1992) and for patients with osteoarthritis (Fisher & Pendergast, 1994). General immune function was improved (Keast & Morton, 1992; Mazzeo & Nasrullah, 1992), as were specific immune functions to ward off infections (Nieman & Nehlsen-Cannarella, 1992) and to increase natural immunity to cancer (Hoffman-Goetz & MacNeil, 1992). Aerobic training also provided considerable benefits after cancer surgery and during chemotherapy (MacVicar & Winningham, 1986; MacVicar et al., 1989). The general finding from these studies is that the benefits of exercise decline rapidly if the exercise stops, so it must be sustained as a lifelong endeavor to continue to have the desired effect. The old maxim "use it or lose it" applies to all ages and stages, including chronically ill older adults.

Exercise, strength training, and balance training, especially in combination, have been shown to reverse several effects of frailty and fall-proneness in the very old. The FICSIT clinical trials are a recent cluster of studies that are attempting to show the reversibility of frailty and preventability of falls in the middle-old and old-old (85 and older) population. Early results are very promising (Fiatarone et al., 1993, 1994; Wolf, Kutner, Green, & McNeely, 1993; Wolfson et al., 1993). A meta-analysis of the results of the seven FICSIT trials showed that across the studies, there was a significant decrease in the 1.5 year (median) follow-up fall rates for the subjects, including both the community (n = 2133) and nursing home subjects (n = 295) (Province et al., 1995). There was not adequate power in the meta-analysis to detect a change in the personal injury fall rate. But significant differences in personal injury risk ratios are very difficult to capture even with a large aggregated sample because even highly fall-prone elders only injure themselves on rare occasions.

Perhaps the most novel intervention of the FICSIT trials is Emory University's T'ai Chi Chuan protocol. A T'ai Chi Grand Master is a member of the research team, and the subjects engage in this dynamic exercise twice each week under the Master's direction. Preliminary results showed increased flexibility, balance, and freedom of movement (McNeely, Clements, & Wolf, 1992).

Roberts and colleagues (Roberts, 1989; Roberts & Wykle, 1993) have been successful in showing positive results of balance training and exercise with frail, elderly, community-dwelling and institutionalized fallers. Hogue and Culliman (1993) also succeeded in decreasing some measures of frailty in a rural sample. The best results in preventing falls among frail elders seem to come from the combination of aerobic fitness training, balance and gait-focused work, and strength training. The basic operating principle in this arena is that there is little or no carryover or spread of benefits. To evoke improvement in functioning, each targeted part or system must be worked. That is, aerobic exercise does not improve strength, strength training does not improve fitness, and neither significantly enhances flexibility or balance. So the protocol must include work on all four components plus nutritional enhancements to optimize the functional independence of the targeted group of elders.

Nutrition

Overnutrition, undernutrition, and malnutrition are prevalent among the chronically ill older population, and each of these conditions is a significant risk factor for poor disease control, exacerbations, and disability. Through a nutrition screening initiative for elders, the American Academy of Family Physicians, the American Dietetic Association, and the National Council on the Aging are seeking to make nutritional status recognized as a "vital sign" in the physical assessment process of all physicians and nurses (Cope, 1994). According to this consortium's published guideline, all patients should receive the Level I screen, which includes height, weight, and body mass index (Dwyer, 1991). Those with an abnormal measurement would go on to Level II testing, which includes assessments of variables such as triceps skin folds, midarm circumference, and albumin and cholesterol levels (Cope, 1994).

It is apparent from a wide array of studies that maintaining proper nutrition is complex but essential to the optimum management of chronic illnesses of the elderly. Studies range from those where good nutritional maintenance can decrease risk of immune dysfunctions such as infections or cancer (Chandra, 1992) to those showing significant decreased risk for cardiovascular disease (Posner, Cupples, Franz, & Gagnon, 1993; Singh, Singh, Rastogi, Mani, & Niaz, 1993).

Other groups of investigators have shown that optimizing nutritional intake leads to significant improvements in the management of chronic disease symptoms, prolongation of remission, and improved independent functioning. Proper nutritional intake has been correlated with deceleration in the progression of Alzheimer's Disease, other dementias, and Parkinsonian symptomatology (Bowman, 1992; Pincus & Barry, 1987, 1988; Rosenberg & Miller, 1992). Good nutrition resulted in the prevention or partial reversal of osteoporosis (Madson, 1989; Sardana, 1992; Walden, 1989; White-O'Connor, Sobal, & Muncie, 1989) and in managing symptoms and preventing complications of diseases such as Type II diabetes (Barnard et al., 1992; Searle & Ready, 1991) and chronic obstructive lung disease (COPD) (Lewis, Belman, & Dorr-Uyemura, 1987).

Finally, nutritional supplementation combined with exercise was found to be highly efficacious in reducing frailty in the old-old subjects in the Boston FICSIT clinical trial (Fiatarone et al., 1994). Improvements were noted in muscle strength, gait velocity, stair-climbing power, thigh-muscle mass, and level of spontaneous (self-initiated) activity. These gains were markedly lower in the samples that engaged in the various exercise protocols without the nutritional supplementation.

Promoting a Sense of Well-being

The most diffuse area of research in health promotion lies in the studies about subjective assessment of well-being. Much of the research focused on preexisting states of morale, life satisfaction, happiness, self-image, self-concept, depression, and other conceptually related perceptions or states. Larson (1978) grouped such concepts into the more global concept of subjective well-being. Most of these studies tended to use ex post facto correlational or other descriptive designs. In general, the findings strongly suggest that chronically ill persons who engage in exercise (Daumer & Miller, 1992; Gift & Austin, 1992) or other health-promoting behaviors (Pollock, Christian, & Sands, 1990) experience higher levels of subjective well-being. Other investigators found that chronically ill persons with positive coping styles, as described in the Lazarus and Folkman (1984) theory of stress and coping, reported significant positive relationships between coping and various concepts in the subjective well-being constellation (Downe-Wambolt, 1991; Lee, Graydon, & Ross, 1991).

Another cluster of concepts includes terms such as hardiness, personal control, sense of independence, autonomy, and self-help. Several investigators found that chronically ill elders reported surprisingly positive attitudes about their situations and their power to manage various aspects of them (Burckhardt, Woods, Schultz, & Ziebarth, 1989; Call & Davis, 1989; Cornwell & Schmitt, 1990; Heidrich, 1993; Laborde & Powers, 1985). Negative influences included severity of illness, older age, and uncertainty (Braden, 1990; Nickel, Brown, & Smith, 1990). Additional positive boosts in well-being were provided by social support (Friedman & King, 1994; Lambert, Lambert, Klipple, & Mewshaw, 1989; Riegel, 1989). Even the terminally ill value autonomy and personal control as components of health during the last stage of life (Fryback, 1993; Fryback & Reinert, 1993).

The number of intervention studies dedicated to influencing subjective well-being to promote health was small. The main forms of intervention were patient education programs (Hunter & Hall, 1989; Neuberger, Smith, Black, & Hassanein, 1993), self-help groups or provider-led groups (Braden, 1993; Ruffing-Rahal, 1993, 1994), or both (Felker, 1988; Newman, 1993). While outcomes tended to be especially positive for those who engaged in ongoing self-help-groups, only a small percentage of affected persons are willing to avail themselves of this resource. The vast majority have a variety of reasons to shun the self-help-group movement. Except for Alcoholics Anonymous, Narcotics Anonymous, and self-help groups for spouse abusers, most self-help groups appeal more to women than to men. There is need for in-depth study of this phenomenon; perhaps new models of self-help need to be developed that are appealing to men. Use of self-help groups with ethnic minorities has shown some possible utility (Ochoco & Shimamoto, 1987), and more work with different minority groups merits attention.

Sexual Health Promotion

Probably the most forgotten, avoided, and neglected aspects of health promotion on the part of health professionals vis-à-vis the elderly and the elderly vis-à-vis themselves are sexual expression, sexual intimacy, and sexual intercourse (McCracken, 1988). Nurse practitioners and rehabilitation nurses in particular have been cautioned to do a thorough sexual assessment, to diagnose and seek treatment for abnormalities, and especially to teach older adults and chronically ill older adults about sexual health and normal sexual behavior in old age (Lyder, 1992, 1994; Smedley, 1991).

Steinke (1994) found that community-dwelling elderly men and women possessed about an equal amount of knowledge about sexuality in later adulthood, and that those with significant others were sexually active a mean of four times per month. In nursing home studies, the men tended to be more interested in being sexually active than the women (McCracken, 1988), but lack of a partner and attitudes of the nursing home staff were major deterrents (Lyder, 1994; Nay, 1992). Lyder emphasized the sexual needs of elderly gays and lesbians in nursing homes, and McCracken focused on the normalcy of masturbation for all elders, whether or not they had access to a sexual partner.

Assessing, teaching about sexual practices, dealing with cultural influences (Billhorn, 1994), and encouraging elders with chronic illnesses to be sexually active in ways that do not increase symptoms or distress have been addressed for various groups of chronically ill elders. The chronic illnesses that require some modification of sexual position or practices include: COPD (Hahn, 1989), insulin-dependent diabetes (LeMone, 1993), and coronary artery bypass grafting and ischemic heart disease

(Relf, 1991). Chronically ill elders should be helped to fulfill their sexual needs as long as it is physically possible and personally desirable for them to do so.

Spiritual Development as Health Promotion

The Duke Longitudinal Studies have provided numerous valuable insights and many surprises about normal aging. Koenig, George, and Siegler (1988) found that even educated elders of higher socioeconomic status depended on spirituality and to a lesser extent on religious coping behaviors to deal with stressful life events, personal losses, and chronic illnesses of old age. Spiritual coping strategies (spirituality) included trust and faith in God, private prayer, and help and strength from a higher power (personal sense of God). Religious coping behaviors related to organized religion and included church activities, ministers' help and guidance, support from church friends, and reading the Bible. Miller (1985) found a negative correlation between loneliness and spiritual well-being in both chronically ill and healthy adults. Further, she found no excess loneliness in the chronically ill group compared to the healthy group, but the chronically ill had significantly higher scores in spiritual well-being.

Gurklis and Menke (1988) showed that prayer and trust in God was the top-ranked coping strategy for 68 subjects receiving hemodialysis. Investigators who have studied patients with various metastatic cancers echo the findings about the strong positive relationship between spirituality and coping with stressful events, poor health, vulnerability, powerlessness, and facing death (Herth, 1989; Sodestrom & Martinson, 1987).

Koenig, Kvale, and Ferrel (1988) attempted to assess the contributions of spirituality and religiosity to well-being (morale) independent of the confounding variables of health, financial status, and social support. In their heterogeneous sample of 805 elders, higher spirituality scores correlated with greater overall morale and less agitation, loneliness, and dissatisfaction with life. A regression analysis disclosed that subjective health accounted for 50% of the explained variance (total variance explained was 33.5%), while the other variables contributed as follows: social support = 24%, financial status = 14%, and spiritual/religious well-being = 13%. In this study as in many others, spirituality and religiosity explained more of the variance for women (17%) than for men (10%).

Reed (1991a) found that persons who were in deep distress because of a health problem wanted to have nurses or other health providers listen to their concerns and fears and the concerns of their family members, but they did not expect or want spiritual guidance from that quarter. They did want nurses to offer to call a minister or other cleric.

The ultimate test of health promotion as a way of life comes during the experience of dying. How well one dies is often considered the ultimate test of emotional maturity, self-actualization, and a host of other concepts in adult development. Reed (1986, 1991a, 1991b) has conducted several studies of the "religiousness" and sense of well-being of terminally ill elders and other adults. Interestingly, she focused her early work (1986) on comparing normal healthy persons with persons in the early phase of their terminal illnesses. These subjects were still relatively independent and ambulatory.

In her early work, Reed (1986) used the term "religiousness" to include both the personal (spiritual) and the organized religion aspects of life. The terminally ill group displayed significantly greater "religiousness." As in other studies, the women, in both groups, were much more religious than the men, that is, even in the terminal phase, men were less likely to turn to religious forms of coping. In a subsequent study of hospitalized terminally ill persons, Reed (1987) found the expected high correlation between what she came to call spirituality (the personal aspects distinct from the organized religion behaviors) and subjective well-being in the terminally ill hospitalized subjects. She also found that a significant number of terminally ill subjects, compared to the healthy controls, indicated a recent change toward more spirituality.

Recently, Reed (1991c, 1992, 1993) derived a middle-range theory about self-transcendence during very old age or the terminal life experience at any age. The essence of the theory is that a healthy way to proceed through the terminal stage of life is by expanding the self-boundaries and developing an orientation toward broadened life perspectives and purposes. Spirituality and deepening spiritual development are integral components of the emerging self-transcendence (Reed, 1991c, 1992), but their exact place in the process and their relative importance to successful development of self-transcendence are still under investigation (Reed, 1992, 1993). In conclusion, spirituality and self-transcendence are critical factors in the maintenance of subjective well-being in the old-old and the terminally ill at any age. It is believed this has to do with the connectedness and wholeness of human beings and with the healthy transition from "being" to "not being." This transition is the final, and perhaps greatest, challenge of human life.

DISCUSSION

The human mind, body, and spirit are eminently resilient, adaptable, and recoverable even in oldest age and with chronic debilitating conditions. The majority of studies on any aspect of health promotion in the chronically ill aged indicate that positive outcomes should be expected. In fact, if positive outcomes are not forthcoming, a careful review of every aspect of the intervention is needed, as well as a thorough analysis of the heterogeneity of the sample to determine whether there was a mismatch between the interventions and some subgroup of the sample. Problems with interventions range from the most obvious violations of the intervention to much more subtle problems. One obvious major problem has been underdosing, either by making the intervention too mild or too short. In every form of intervention discussed in this review, the older adults likely will require twice or many times the length of intervention compared to younger persons. In addition, time may be spent overcoming an age-based cohort bias or other negative attitudes toward the intervention by the elders, or time may be spent building up to a therapeutic dose of the intervention. Many elders are so hypokinetic they require 3 or 4 months of mild exercise just to get to a level of work that will raise their pulse to an aerobic fitness level. Likewise, many elders have avoided fiber to such an extent that it could take up to a year to raise them to the daily level recommended by nutritionists without causing severe gas pains, cramping, and diarrhea. Or in a progressive relaxation-guided imagery protocol, they may take extra time learning the procedure before they can practice it properly and even begin to derive the benefits.

Many elders have not stretched their cognitive abilities or tried to improve their memories for decades; hence cognitive interventions may take an extended period of time, and considerable coaching and encouragement may be needed to foster the proper motivation to stick with the program. For health promotion to work in an optimum fashion, first, it is necessary that the subjects be motivated—that is, they must have faith in the outcomes, desire the outcomes, and be willing to work for the outcomes. Second, it is essential that the intervention protocol be designed just right—that is, it must not be too strong or too weak, it must be lengthy enough, and it must be an excellent match with the abilities and needs of the subjects.

Third, the sample must be homogeneously matched to the protocol—that is, the group must not contain elders who need a different kind of protocol or a different level of the protocol. An example of this last point would be to implement a chair exercise protocol with a group of elders that included individuals who belong in a more strenuous treadmill/bicycle ergometer and weight-machine training program. Nobody benefits from mismatching the subjects with the treatment. Some elders will be bored, some may be harmed by overreaching their capacity, results will be attenuated, false conclusions can be reached, the staff could become disillusioned, and future ventures into health-promoting activity might be stifled.

Fourth, the metaintervention must be carefully developed and orchestrated. The components of the metaintervention may include:

1. the introduction to the program—the sales pitch and explanation of the activity and the expected benefits;
2. the instructions about what to do, when, and how—elders may have sensory deficits or poor memory habits and require multiple modes of explanation, several repetitions, and close supervision and coaching;
3. the equipment should be simple, the explanations of its use must be simple, the proper use of the equipment should be demonstrated, and the explanations or directions ought to be repeated each time the equipment is used; and
4. the environment or site of the intervention must be optimized. Criteria for appropriate sites include a quiet place with adequate space for the program and proper temperature and humidity to encourage the activity.

Even a nutrition intervention will work better in a nice environment that is conducive to experimenting with new foods. Interventions in the realm of sexual health promotion or spiritual health promotion are very sensitive to the quality of the environment, and privacy is generally a must.

Planning and facilitating health-promotion programs for chronically ill older adults are not for the impatient or weak of heart. Establishing such programs is an exceedingly challenging and demanding undertaking. However, the rewards are well worth the effort, and, with practice, the necessary patience is learned and the slower pacing of activities becomes second nature. The major impediment to health promotion for chronically ill elders among the nursing and health care community is ageism and lack of faith that health promotion can or will have discernible, positive outcomes. Only time, experience, and modeling of successes will overcome an unfortunate impediment to this highly challenging and rewarding aspect of gerontological care.

REFERENCES

Adamopoulos, S., Coats, A. J. S., Brunotte, F., Arnolda, L., Meyer, T., Thompson, C. H., Dunn, J. F., Stratton, J., Kemp, G. J., Radda, G. K., & Rajagopalan, B. (1993). Physical training improves skeletal muscle metabolism in patients with chronic heart failure. *Journal of the American College of Cardiology, 21*(5), 1101–1106.

Agre, J. C., Pierce, L. E., Raab, D. M., McAdams, M., & Smith, E. L. (1988). Light resistance and stretching exercise in elderly women: Effect upon strength. *Archives of Physical Medicine and Rehabilitation, 69*(4), 273–276.

Alderman, M. H. (1994). Non-pharmacological treatment of hypertension. *Lancet, 344*(5), 307–311.

Balady, G. J. (1992). Exercise therapy in patients with angina and silent ischemia. In R. J. Shepard & H. S. Miller, Jr. (Eds.), *Exercise and the heart in health and disease* (pp. 369–396). New York: Marcel Dekker.

Barnard, R. J., Ugianskis, E. J., & Martin, D. A. (1992). The effects of an intensive diet and exercise program on patients with non-insulin-dependent diabetes mellitus and hypertension. *Journal of Cardiopulmonary Rehabilitation, 12*(3), 194–201.

Berry, E. M. (1994). Chronic disease: How can nutrition moderate the effects? *Nutrition Reviews, 52*(8), S28–S30.

Billhorn, D. R. (1994). Sexuality and the chronically ill older adult: What can nursing do to assist the chronically ill older adult to recognize and fulfill feelings of sexuality? *Geriatric Nursing, 15*(2), 106–108.

Black, J. S., & Kapoor, W. (1990). Health promotion and disease prevention in older people: Our current state of ignorance. *Journal of the American Geriatrics Society, 38*(2), 168–172.

Blair, S. N., Kohl, H. W., III., Paffenbarger, R. S., Jr., Clark, D. G., Cooper, K. H., & Gibbons, L. W. (1989). Physical fitness and all-cause mortality: A prospective study of healthy men and women. *Journal of the American Medical Association, 262*(17), 2395–2401.

Blumenthal, J. A., Emery, C. F., Madden, D. J., George, L. K., Coleman, R. E., Riddle, M. W., McKee, D. C., Reasoner, J., & Williams, R. S. (1989). Cardiovascular and behavioral effects of aerobic exercise training in healthy older men and women. *Journal of Gerontology, 44*(5), 147–157.

Blumenthal, J. A., Siegel, W. C., & Applebaum, M. (1991). Failure of exercise to reduce blood pressure in patients with mild hypertension: Results of a controlled clinical trial. *Journal of the American Medical Association, 266*(15), 2098–2100.

Bonnel, W. B. (1993). Cognitive control: A concept worth considering for older adult clients. *Kansas Nurse, 68*(6), 4–5.

Bowman, B. A. B. (1992). Acetyl-carnitine and Alzheimer's disease. *Nutrition Reviews, 50*(5), 142–144.

Braden, C. J. (1993). Promoting a learned self-help response to chronic illness. In S. G. Funk, E. M. Tornquist, M. T. Champagne, & R. A. Wiese (Eds.), *Key aspects of caring for the chronically ill: Hospital and home* (pp. 158–169). New York: Springer.

Braden, C. J. (1990). A test of the self-help model: Learned response to chronic illness experience. *Nursing Research, 39*(1), 42–47.

Buchner, D. M., & Wagner, E. H. (1992). Preventing frail health. *Clinics in Geriatric Medicine, 8*(1), 1–17.

Burckhardt, C. S., Woods, S. L., Schultz, A. A., & Ziebarth, D. M. (1989). Quality of life of adults with chronic illness: A psychometric study. *Research in Nursing and Health, 12*(6), 347–354.

Call, J. G., & Davis, L. L. (1989). The effect of hardiness on coping strategies and adjustment to illness in chronically ill individuals. *Applied Nursing Research, 2*(4), 187–188.

Chandra, R. K. (1992). Effect of vitamin and trace-element supplementation on immune responses and infection in elderly subjects. *Lancet, 340*(8828), 1124–1127.

Collison, C., & Miller, S. (1987). Using images of the future in grief work. *Image: Journal of Nursing Scholarship, 19*(1), 9–11.

Cope, K. A. (1994). Nutritional status: A basic "vital sign." *Home Healthcare Nurse, 12*(2), 29–34.

Cornwell, C. J., & Schmitt, M. H. (1990). Perceived health status, self-esteem and body image in women with rheumatoid arthritis or systemic lupus erythematosus. *Research in Nursing and Health, 13*(2), 99–107.

Daumer, R., & Miller, P. (1992). Effects of cardiac rehabilitation on psychosocial functioning and life satisfaction of coronary artery disease clients. *Rehabilitation Nursing, 17*(2), 69–75.

Diesfeldt, H. F. A., & Diesfeldt-Groenendijk, H. (1977). Improving cognitive performance in psychogeriatric patients: The influence of physical exercise. *Aging, 6,* 58–64.

Downe-Wambolt, B. (1991). Coping and life satisfaction in elderly women with osteoarthritis. *Journal of Advanced Nursing, 16*(11), 1328–1335.

Duffy, M. E. (1993). Determinants of health-promoting lifestyles in older persons. *Image: Journal of Nursing Scholarship, 25*(1), 23–28.

Dustman, R. E., Ruhling, R. O., Russell, E. M., Shearer, D. E., Bonekat, H. W., Shigeoka, J. W., Wood, J. A., & Bradford, D. C. (1984). Aerobic exercise training and improved neuropsychological function of older individuals. *Neurobiology of Aging, 5*(1), 35–42.

Dwyer, J. T. (1991). *Nutrition screening I: Toward a common view.* Washington, DC: Nutrition Screening Initiative.

Felker, M. P. (1988). A recovery group for elderly alcoholics. *Geriatric Nursing, 9*(2), 110–113.

Ferraro, K. F. (1993). Are black older adults health-pessimistic? *Journal of Health and Social Behavior, 34*(3), 201–214.

Fiatarone, M. A., Marks, E. C., Ryan, N. D., Meredith, C. N., Lipsitz, L. A., & Evans, W. J. (1990). High-intensity strength training in nonagenarians: Effects on skeletal muscle. *Journal of the American Medical Association, 263*(22), 3029–3034.

Fiatarone, M. A., O'Neill, E. F., Doyle, N., Clements, K. M., Roberts, S. B., Kehayias, J. J., Lipsitz, L. A., & Evans, W. J. (1993). The Boston FICSIT study: The effects of resistance training and nutritional supplementation on physical frailty in the oldest old. *Journal of the American Geriatrics Society, 41*(3), 333–337.

Fiatarone, M. A., O'Neill, E. F., Ryan, N. D., Clements, K. M., Solares, G. R., Nelson, M. E., Roberts, S. B., Kehayias, J. J., Lipsitz, L. A., & Evans, W. J. (1994). Exercise training and nutritional supplementation for physical frailty in very elderly people. *New England Journal of Medicine, 330*(25), 1769–1775.

Fisher, N. M., Kame, V. D., Rouse, L., & Pendergast, D. R. (1994). Quantitative evaluation of a home exercise program on muscle and functional capacity of patients with osteoarthritis. *American Journal of Physical Medicine and Rehabilitation, 73*(6), 413–420.

Fisher, N. M., & Pendergast, D. R. (1994). Effects of a muscle exercise program on exercise capacity in subjects with osteoarthritis. *Archives of Physical Medicine and Rehabilitation, 75*(7), 792–797.

Fisher, N. M., Pendergast, D. R., & Calkins, E. (1991). Muscle rehabilitation in impaired elderly nursing home residents. *Archives of Physical Medicine and Rehabilitation, 72*, 181–185.

Fletcher, B. J., & Vassallo, L. M. (1993). Exercise testing and training in physically disabled subjects with coronary artery disease. In S. G. Funk, E. M. Tornquist, M. T. Champagne, & R. A. Wiese (Eds.), *Key aspects of caring for the chronically ill: Hospital and home* (pp. 189–201). New York: Springer.

Foster, C., & Tamboli, H. P. (1992). Exercise prescription in the rehabilitation of patients following coronary artery bypass graft surgery and coronary angioplasty. In R. J. Shepard & H. S. Miller, Jr. (Eds.), *Exercise and the heart in health and disease* (pp. 283–298). Boca Raton, FL: Marcel Dekker.

Foster, M. F. (1992). Health promotion and life satisfaction in elderly black adults. *Western Journal of Nursing Research, 14*(4), 444–463.

Friedman, M. M., & King, K. B. (1994). The relationship of emotional and tangible support to psychological well-being among older women with heart failure. *Research in Nursing and Health, 17*(6), 433–440.

Fryback, P. B. (1993). Health for people with a terminal diagnosis. *Nursing Science Quarterly, 6*(3), 147–159.

Fryback, P. B., & Reinert, B. R. (1993). Facilitating health in people with terminal diagnoses by encouraging a sense of control. *Medsurg Nursing, 2*(3), 197–201.

Gift, A. G., & Austin, D. J. (1992). The effects of a program of systematic movement on COPD patients. *Rehabilitation Nursing, 17*(1), 6–10.

Gurklis, J. A., & Menke, E. M. (1988). Identification of stressors and use of coping methods in chronic hemodialysis patients. *Nursing Research, 37*(4), 236–248.

Hahn, K. (1989). Sexuality and COPD. *Rehabilitation Nursing, 14*(4), 191–195.

Hahn, Y. B., Ro, Y. J., Song, H. H., Kim, N. C., Kim, H. S., & Yoo, Y. S. (1993). The effect of thermal biofeedback and progressive relaxation training in reducing blood pressure of patients with essential hypertension. *Image: Journal of Nursing Scholarship, 25*(3), 204–207.

Hall, N., De Beck, P., Johnson, P., & Mackinnon, R. (1992). Randomized trial of health promotion for frail elders. *Canadian Journal of Aging, 11,* 72–91.

Heidrich, S. M. (1993). The relationship between physical and psychological well-being in elderly women: A developmental perspective. *Research in Nursing and Health, 16*(2), 123–130.

Herth, K. A. (1989). The relationship between level of hope and level of coping response and other variables in patients with cancer. *Oncology Nursing Forum, 16*(1), 67–72.

Hoffman-Goetz, L., & MacNeil, B. (1992). Exercise, natural immunity, and cancer: Causation, correlation, or conundrum. In R. R. Watson & M. Eisinger (Eds.), *Exercise and disease* (pp. 37–62). Boca Raton, FL: CRC Press.

Hogue, C. C., & Culliman, S. M. (1993). Exercise training for frail rural elderly: A pilot study. In S. G. Funk, E. M. Tornquist, M. T. Champagne, & R. A. Wiese (Eds.), *Key aspects of caring for the chronically ill: Hospital and home* (pp. 202–211). New York: Springer.

Howell, S. L. (1994). Natural/alternative health care practices used by women with chronic pain: Findings from a grounded theory research study. *Nurse Practitioner Forum, 5*(2), 98–105.

Hunter, S. M., & Hall, S. S. (1989). The effect of an educational support program on dyspnea and the emotional status of COPD clients. *Rehabilitation Nursing, 14*(4), 200–202.

Jirovec, M. M. (1991). The impact of daily exercise on the mobility, balance and urine control of cognitively impaired nursing home residents. *International Journal of Nursing Studies, 28*(2), 145–151.

Kane, R. L., Ouslander, J. G., & Abrass, I. B. (1994). *Essentials of clinical geriatrics* (3rd ed.). New York: McGraw-Hill.

Kaplun, A. (Ed.). (1992). *Health promotion and chronic illness: Discovering a new quality of health.* Copenhagen: World Health Association.

Kavanagh, T. (1992). Exercise and therapy of the cardiac transplant patients. In R. J. Shepard & H. S. Miller, Jr. (Eds.), *Exercise and the heart in health and disease* (pp. 257–282). New York: Marcel Dekker.

Keast, D., & Morton, A. R. (1992). Long-term exercise and immune function. In R. R. Watson & M. Eisinger (Eds.), *Exercise and disease* (pp. 89–120). Boca Raton, FL: CRC Press.

Kim, M. J., Larson, J. L., Covey, M. K., Vitalo, C. A., Alex, C. G., & Patel, M. (1993). Inspiratory muscle training in patients with chronic obstructive pulmonary disease. *Nursing Research, 42*(6), 356–362.

Koenig, H. G., George, L. K., & Siegler, I. C. (1988). The use of religion and other emotion-regulating coping strategies among older adults. *Gerontologist, 28*(3), 303–310.

Koenig, H. G., Kvale, J. N., & Ferrel, C. (1988). Religion and well-being in later life. *Gerontologist, 28*(1), 18–28.

Kotthoff-Burrell, E. (1992). Health promotion and disease prevention for the older adult: An overview of the current recommendations and a practical application. *Nurse Practitioner Forum, 3*(4), 195–209.

Laborde, J. M., & Powers, M. J. (1985). Life satisfaction, health control orientation, and illness-related factors in persons with osteoarthritis. *Research in Nursing and Health, 8*(2), 183–190.

Lambert, V. A., Lambert, C. E., Klipple, G. L., & Mewshaw, E. A. (1989). Social support, hardiness and psychological well-being in women with arthritis. *Image: Journal of Nursing Scholarship, 21*(3), 128–131.

Larson, R. (1978). Thirty years of research on the subjective well-being of older Americans. *Journal of Gerontology, 33*, 109–125.

Lauder, W. (1993). Health promotion in the elderly. *British Journal of Nursing, 2*(8), 401–404.

Lazarus, R. S., & Folkman, S. (1984). *Stress, appraisal, and coping.* New York: Springer.

Lee, R. N. F., Graydon, J. E., & Ross, E. (1991). Effects of psychological well-being, physical status, and social support on oxygen-dependent COPD patients' level of functioning. *Research in Nursing and Health, 14*(5), 323–329.

LeMone, P. (1993). Human sexuality in adults with insulin-dependent diabetes mellitus. *Image: Journal of Nursing Scholarship, 25*(2), 101–105.

Leon, A. S. (1992). The role of exercise in the prevention and management of diabetes mellitus and blood lipid disorders. In R. J. Shepard & H. S. Miller, Jr. (Eds.), *Exercise and the heart in health and disease* (pp. 299–368). Boca Raton, FL: Marcel Dekker.

Lesko, W. A., & Summerfield, L. M. (1988). The effectiveness of biofeedback and home relaxation training on reduction of borderline hypertension. *Health Education, 19*(5), 19–23.

Lewis, M. I., Belman, M. J., & Dorr-Uyemura, L. (1987). Nutritional supplementation in ambulatory patients with chronic obstructive pulmonary disease. *American Review of Respiratory Disease, 135*(5), 1062–1068.

Lindenmuth, G. F., & Moose, B. (1990). Improving cognitive abilities of elderly Alzheimer's patients with intense exercise therapy. *American Journal of Alzheimer's Care and Related Disorders & Research, 1,* 31–33.

Lyder, C. H. (1992). NPs play major role in promoting sexuality among institutionalized elderly [Letter to the editor]. *Nurse Practitioner: American Journal of Primary Health, 17*(9), 10, 13.

Lyder, C. H. (1994). The role of the nurse practitioner in promoting sexuality in the institutionalized elderly. *Journal of the American Academy of Nurse Practitioners, 6*(2), 61–63.

Mace, N. L. (1987). Principles of activities for persons with dementia. *Physical and Occupational Therapy in Geriatrics, 5*(3), 13–27.

MacVicar, M. G., & Winningham, M. L. (1986). Promoting the functional capacity of cancer patients. *Cancer Bulletin, 38,* 235.

MacVicar, M. G., Winningham, M. L., & Nickel, J. L. (1989). Effects of aerobic interval training on cancer patients' functional capacity. *Nursing Research, 38(6)*, 348–351.

Madson, S. (1989). How to reduce risk of postmenopausal osteoporosis. *Journal of Gerontological Nursing, 15*(9), 77–78, 83, 84.

Mazzeo, R. S., & Nasrullah, I. (1992). Exercise and age-related decline in immune functions. In R. R. Watson & M. Eisinger (Eds.), *Exercise and disease* (pp. 159–178). Boca Raton, FL: CRC Press.

McCracken, A. L. (1988). Sexual practice by elders: The forgotten aspect of functional health. *Journal of Gerontological Nursing, 14*(10), 13–18.

McEwan, R. T., Davison, N., Forster, D. P., Pearson, P., & Stirling, E. (1990). Screening elderly people in primary care: A randomized control trial. *British Journal of General Practice, 40*(332), 94–97.

McMurdo, M. E., & Rennie, L. (1993). A controlled trial of exercise by residents of old people's homes. *Age and Ageing, 22,* 11–15.

McNeely, E., Clements, S. D., & Wolf, S. L. (1992). A program to reduce frailty in the elderly. In S. G. Funk, E. M. Tornquist, M. T. Champagne, & R. A. Wiese (Eds.), *Key aspects of elder care: Managing falls, incontinence, and cognitive impairment* (pp. 89–96). New York: Springer.

Miller, H. S., Jr., & Paffenbarger, R. S., Jr. (1992). The prevention and treatment of coronary disease: The case for exercise. In R. J. Shepard & H. S. Miller, Jr. (Eds.), *Exercise and the heart in health and disease* (pp. 251–256). New York: Marcel Dekker.

Miller, J. F. (1985). Assessment of loneliness and spiritual well-being in chronically ill and healthy adults. *Journal of Professional Nursing, 1*(2), 79–85.

Miller, M. P. (1991). Factors promoting wellness in the aged person: An ethnographic study. *Advances in Nursing Science, 13*(4), 38–51.

Milz, H. (1992). "Healthy ill people": Social cynicism or new perspectives? In A. Kaplun (Ed.), *Health promotion and chronic illness: Discovering a new quality of health* (pp. 32–39). Copenhagen: World Health Organization.

Molloy, D. W., Beerschoten, D. A., Borrie, M. J., Crilly, R. G., & Cape, R. D. T. (1988). Acute effects of exercise on neuropsychological function in elderly subjects. *Journal of the American Geriatrics Society, 36*(1), 29–33.

Molloy, D. W., Richardson, L. D., & Crilly, R. G. (1988). The effects of a three-month exercise programme on neuropsychological function in elderly institutionalized women: A randomized controlled trial. *Age and Ageing, 17*(5), 303–310.

Moody, L. E., Fraser, M., & Yarandi, H. (1993). Effects of guided imagery in patients with chronic bronchitis and emphysema. *Clinical Nursing Research, 2*(4), 478–486.

Morey, M. C., Crowley, G. M., Robbins, M. S., Cowper, P. A., & Sullivan, R. J., Jr. (1994). The Gerofit program: A VA innovation. *Southern Medical Journal, 87*(5), S83–S87.

Nay, R. (1992). Sexuality and aged women in nursing homes. *Geriatric Nursing, 13*(6), 312–314.

Nelson, M. E., Fiatarone, M. A., Morganti, C. M., Trice, I., Greenberg, R. A., & Evans, W. J. (1994). Effects of high-intensity strength training on multiple risk factors for osteoporotic fractures: A randomized controlled trial. *Journal of the American Medical Association, 272*(24), 1909–1914.

Neuberger, G. B., Smith, K. V., Black, S. O., & Hassanein, R. (1993). Promoting self-care in clients with arthritis. *Arthritis Care and Research, 6*(3), 141–148.

Newman, A. M. (1993). Effect of a self-help course on adaptation in people with arthritis. In S. G. Funk, E. M. Tornquist, M. T. Champagne, & R. A. Wiese (Eds.), *Key aspects of caring for the chronically ill: Hospital and home* (pp. 150–157). New York: Springer.

Nickel, J. T., Brown, K. J., & Smith, B. A. (1990). Depression and anxiety among chronically ill heart patients: Age differences in risk and predictors. *Research in Nursing and Health, 13*(2), 87–97.

Nieman, D. C., & Nehlsen-Cannarella, S. L. (1992). Exercise and infection. In R. R. Watson & M. Eisinger (Eds.), *Exercise and disease* (pp. 121–148). Boca Raton, FL: CRC Press.

Ochoco, L., & Shimamoto, Y. (1987). Group work with the frail ethnic elderly. *Geriatric Nursing, 8*(4), 185–187.

O'Connor, G. T., Buring, J. E., Yusuf, S., Goldhaber, S. Z., Olmstead, E. M., Paffenbarger, R. S., Jr., & Hennekens, C. H. (1989). An overview of randomized trials of rehabilitation with exercise after myocardial infarction. *Circulation, 80*(2), 234–244.

Pender, N. J. (1982). *Health promotion in nursing practice.* Norwalk, CT: Appleton-Century-Crofts.

Perri, S., & Templer, D. I. (1985). The effects of an aerobic exercise program on psychological variables in older adults. *International Journal of Aging and Human Development, 20*(3), 167–172.

Pincus, J., & Barry, K. (1987). Plasma levels of amino acids correlate with motor fluctuations in Parkinsonism. *Archives of Neurology, 44*(10), 1006–1009.

Pincus, J., & Barry, K. (1988). Protein redistribution diet restores motor function in patients with dopa-resistant "off" periods. *Neurology, 38*(3), 481–483.

Pollock, S. E., Christian, B. J., & Sands, D. (1990). Responses to chronic illness: Analysis of psychological and physiological adaptation. *Nursing Research, 39*(5), 300–304.

Posner, B. M., Cupples, L. A., Franz, M. M., & Gagnon, D. R. (1993). Diet and heart disease risk factors in adult American men and women: The Framingham offspring-spouse nutrition studies. *International Journal of Epidemiology, 22*(6), 1014–1025.

Province, M. A., Hadley, E. C., Hornbrook, M. C., Lipsitz, L. A., Miller, J. P., Mulrow, C. D., Ory, M. G., Sattin, R. W., Tinetti, M. E., & Wolf, S. L. (1995). The effects of exercise on falls in elderly patients: A preplanned meta-analysis of the FICSIT trials. *Journal of the American Medical Association, 273*(17), 1341–1347.

Radecki, S. E., & Mendenhall, R. C. (1986). Patient counseling by primary care physicians: Results of a nationwide survey. *Patient Education Counseling, 8,* 165–177.

Reed, P. G. (1986). Religiousness among terminally ill and healthy adults. *Research in Nursing and Health, 9*(1), 35–41.

Reed, P. G. (1987). Spirituality and well-being in terminally ill hospitalized adults. *Research in Nursing and Health, 10*(5), 335–344.

Reed, P. G. (1991a). Preferences for spiritually related nursing interventions among terminally ill and nonterminally ill hospitalized adults and well adults. *Applied Nursing Research, 4*(3), 122–128.

Reed, P. G. (1991b). Self-transcendence and mental health in oldest-old adults. *Nursing Research, 40*(1), 5–11.

Reed, P. G. (1991c). Toward a nursing theory of self-transcendence: Deductive reformulation using developmental theories. *ANS—Advances in Nursing Science, 13*(4), 64–77.

Reed, P. G. (1992). An emerging paradigm for the investigation of spirituality in nursing. *Research in Nursing and Health, 15*(5), 349–357.

Reed, P. G. (1993, June). *Identifying the critical phenomena of nursing itself—Innate developmental processes of health.* Paper presented at the Annual Forum for Doctoral Nursing Education, St. Paul, MN.

Relf, M. V. (1991). Sexuality and the older bypass patient. *Geriatric Nursing, 12*(6), 294–296.

Renfroe, K. L. (1988). Effect of progressive relaxation on dyspnea and state anxiety in patients with chronic obstructive pulmonary disease. *Heart & Lung: Journal of Critical Care, 17*(4), 408–413.

Richardson, J. P. (1992). Health promotion for the nursing home patient. *Journal of the American Board of Family Practice, 5*(2), 127–136.

Riegel, B. (1989). Social support and psychological adjustment to chronic coronary heart disease: Operationalization of Johnson's behavioral system model. *Advances in Nursing Science, 11*(2), 74–84.

Roberts, B. L. (1989). Effects of walking on balance among elders. *Nursing Research, 38*(3), 180–182.

Roberts, B. L., & Algase, D. L. (1988). Victims of Alzheimer's disease and the environment. *Nursing Clinics of North America, 23*(1), 83–93.

Roberts, B. L., & Lincoln, R. E. (1988). Cognitive disturbance in hospitalized and institutionalized elders. *Research in Nursing and Health, 11*(5), 309–319.

Roberts, B. L., & Wykle, M. L. (1993). Pilot study results: Falls among institutionalized elderly. *Journal of Gerontological Nursing, 19*(5), 13–20.

Robertson, J. F. (1991). Promoting health among the institutionalized elderly. *Journal of Gerontological Nursing, 17*(6), 15–19.

Rosenberg, I. H., & Miller, J. W. (1992). Nutritional factors in physical and cognitive functions of elderly people. *American Journal of Clinical Nutrition, 55*(Suppl. 6), 1237S–1243S.

Rosling, L. K., & Kitchen, J. (1992). Music and drawing with institutionalized elderly. *Activities, Adaptation and Aging, 17*(2), 27–38.

Rubenstein, L. Z., Aronow, H. U., Schloe, M., Steiner, A., Alessi, C. A., Yuhas, K. E., Gold, M., Kemp, M., Raube, K., Nisenbaum, R., Stuck, A., & Beck, J. C. (1994). A home-based geriatric assessment, follow-up and health promotion program: Design, methods, and baseline findings from a 3-year randomized clinical trial. *Aging, 6*(2), 105–120.

Ruffing-Rahal, M. A. (1993). An ecological model of group well-being: Implications for health promotion with older women. *Health Care for Women International, 14*(5), 447–456.

Ruffing-Rahal, M. A. (1994). Evaluation of group health promotion with community dwelling older women. *Public Health Nursing, 11*(1), 38–48.

Russell, N. K., & Roter, D. L. (1993). Health promotion counseling of chronic-disease patients during primary care visits. *American Journal of Public Health, 83*(7), 979–982.

Sardana, R. (1992). Nutritional management of osteoporosis. To slow the advancement of osteoporosis, nurses must encourage their clients to increase their intake of calcium. For geriatric nurses, this may be a challenge. *Geriatric Nursing, 14*(2), 315–319.

Sauvage, L. R., Myklebust, B. M., Crow-Pan, J., Novak, S., Millington, P., Hoffman, M. D., Hartz, A. J., & Rudman, D. (1992). A clinical trial of strengthening and aerobic exercise to improve gait and balance in elderly male nursing home residents. *Journal of Physical Medicine and Rehabilitation, 71*(6), 333–342.

Schorr, J. A. (1993). Music and pattern change in chronic pain. *Advances in Nursing Science, 15*(4), 27–36.

Searle, M. S., & Ready, A. E. (1991). Survey of exercise and dietary knowledge and behaviour in persons with type II diabetes. *Canadian Journal of Public Health, 82*(5), 344–348.

Singh, R. B., Singh, N. K., Rastogi, S. S., Mani, U. V, & Niaz, M. A. (1993). Effects of diet and lifestyle changes on atherosclerotic risk factors after 24 weeks on the Indian diet heart study. *American Journal of Cardiology, 71*(1), 1283–1288.

Slivinske, L., & Fitch, V. (1987). The effect of control enhancing interventions on the well-being of elderly individuals living in retirement communities. *Gerontologist, 27*(2), 176–181.

Smedley, G. (1991). Addressing sexuality in the elderly. *Rehabilitation Nursing, 16*(1), 9–11.

Smith, L. K. (1992). Exercise in patients with heart failure. In R. J. Shepard & H. S. Miller, Jr. (Eds.), *Exercise and the heart in health and disease* (pp. 397–412). Boca Raton, FL: Marcel Dekker.

Sodestrom, K. E., & Martinson, I. M. (1987). Patients' spiritual coping strategies: A study of nurse and patient perspectives. *Oncology Nursing Forum, 14*(2), 41–46.

Stamford, B. A. (1988). Exercise and the elderly. *Exercise and Sports Sciences Reviews, 16,* 341–379.

Steinke, E. E. (1994). Knowledge and attitudes of older adults about sexuality in ageing: A comparison of two studies. *Journal of Advanced Nursing, 19*(3), 477–485.

Stevenson, J. S. (1988). *Effects of preventive exercise in frail elders* (Final Rep. No. RF717732). Columbus, OH: Ohio State University Research Foundation.

Stevenson, J. S., & Topp, R. (1990). Effects of moderate and low intensity long-term exercise by older adults. *Research in Nursing and Health, 13*(4), 209–218.

Stuck, A. E., Mayer-Oakes, A., & Rubenstein, L. Z. (1993). Geriatric in-home preventive programs: Facts and challenges. *L'Année Gérontologique, 7,* 357–365.

Stuifbergen, A. K., & Becker, H. A. (1994). Predictors of health promoting lifestyles in persons with disabilities. *Research in Nursing and Health, 17*(1), 3–13.

Topp, R., & Stevenson, J. S. (1994). The effects of attendance and effort on outcomes among older adults in a long-term exercise program. *Research in Nursing and Health, 17*(1), 15–24.

Valentine-Garzon, M. A., Maynard, M., & Selznick, S. Z. (1992). ROM dance program effects on frail elderly women in an adult day-care program. *Physical & Occupational Therapy in Geriatrics, 11*(1), 63–83.

Verbrugge, L. M., Lepkowski, J. M., & Imanaka, Y. (1989). Comorbidity and its impact on disability. *Milbank Memorial Fund Quarterly, 67*(3–4), 450–484.

Walden, O. (1989). The relationship of dietary and supplemental calcium intake to bone loss and osteoporosis. *Journal of the American Dietetics Association, 89*(3), 397–400.

Walker, S. N., Sechrist, K. R., & Pender, N. J. (1987). The Health-Promoting Lifestyle Profile: Development and psychometric characteristics. *Nursing Research, 36*(2), 76–81.

Wechsler, H., Levine, S., Idelson, R. K., Rohman, M., & Taylor, J. O. (1983). The physician's role in health promotion: A survey of primary care practitioners. *New England Journal of Medicine, 308,* 97–100.

Whetstone, W. R., & Reid, J. C. (1991). Health promotion of older adults: Perceived barriers. *Journal of Advanced Nursing, 16*(11), 1343–1349.

White-O'Connor, B., Sobal, J., & Muncie, H. L., Jr. (1989). Dietary habits, weight history, and vitamin supplement use in elderly osteoarthritis patients. *Journal of the American Dietetic Association, 89*(3), 378–382.

Wolf, S. L., Kutner, N. G., Green, R. C., & McNeely, E. (1993). The Atlanta FICSIT study: Two exercise interventions to reduce frailty in elders. *Journal of the American Geriatrics Society, 41*(3), 329–332.

Wolfson, L., Whipple, R., Judge, J., Amerman, P., Derby, C., & King, M. (1993). Training balance and strength in the elderly to improve function. *Journal of the American Geriatrics Society, 41*(3), 341–343.

CHAPTER 3

Caring for the Aged in the Community

Juliet M. Corbin and Julie C. Cherry

> You know when you get old, nobody pays attention to you. They say all your problems [medical] are due to age and there is nothing they can do. They say, "What can you expect at your age?" You just have to live with it (personal communication, May 10, 1995).

Those of us working with older adults know that their medical problems are very real. These problems cannot be attributed solely to age, but are often the result of chronic conditions, the incidence of which tends to increase with age (National Center for Health Statistics, 1992). Furthermore, there is something that can be done. Those chronically ill older adults who are able to keep their medical conditions stable are more likely to remain living independently and to have genuine quality of life than those who suffer from disabling chronic conditions and their complications. In fact, the chronically ill try to normalize their lives as much as possible (Robinson, 1993), although the task of normalizing can be very difficult when symptoms and complications keep intruding into life's activities.

Chronic illnesses and their complications are a major problem of elders. The management of those conditions takes place mainly in the home. It is here that daily regimens are carried out to keep the illness conditions stable. Stability means fewer complications and symptoms to intrude upon life, therefore, greater quality of life. Keeping a chronic illness stable is not an easy task. It is a complex process that requires the ability to: (a) implement regimens, (b) monitor signs of complications and symptoms, (c) manage disabilities, and (d) come to terms with psychosocial responses to illness and disability (Corbin & Strauss, 1988). Psychosocial responses include but are not limited to: (a) social isolation, (b) financial hardships, (c) the constriction of time, (d) identity insults, and (e) a profound sense of loss (Charmaz, 1983; Strauss & Glaser, 1975).

It is not uncommon for older persons to have more than one chronic condition. Between the ages of 70 and 79, 61% of the population will experience two or more chronic conditions. Comorbidity jumps to 70% by the age of 80 (Guralnik, LaCroix, Everett, & Kovar, 1989). The presence of multiple chronic conditions can mean having several medical regimens to follow, with an increased potential for adverse drug reactions and interactions (Colley & Lucas, 1993; Gambert, Grossberg, & Morley, 1994). In addition, carrying out regimens is time consuming. Some chronically ill elders complain that much of their day is spent carrying out regimens, leaving little time or energy for more fulfilling activities. Then, too, those elders with limited resources find it difficult to pay for expensive drugs or to purchase the equipment and services that might facilitate illness and disability management.

Complicating older persons' ability to manage their chronic conditions are the normal physiological changes that come with aging. These include: declining vision and hearing, decreased energy and mobility, and dexterity limitations (Kane, Ouslander, & Abrass, 1994). All or any of these may impair older persons' ability to follow treatment instructions as prescribed, and also increase the possibility of their making medication errors.

Although the problems of managing chronic illness are complex and varied, to say to an older person that "nothing can be done" and "you just have to live with it" is wrong! With proper support and management, elders can be helped to keep their chronic conditions stable or to regain stability following complications. It is possible for them to have considerable quality of life despite aging and illness. Then, when the time comes, they can be given the support needed to die with dignity (Strauss & Corbin, 1988).

This chapter focuses on an elderly population living independently in the community. There are four sections to the chapter. The first section explains why some older adults become part of a population at risk. The second section provides an overview of the Corbin and Strauss Chronic Illness Trajectory Framework (Corbin & Strauss, 1991; Woog, 1992), a model that can be used to contain those risks. The third section presents an overview of community-based models of care and describes how nurse-managed centers fit within that larger picture of community-based models. The fourth section explains, using case illustrations, how the Corbin and Strauss Chronic Illness Trajectory Framework has been used in one nurse-managed center to reduce the problems that arise from inadequate medical care and social services and to enhance the quality of life.

A POPULATION AT RISK

Although it is often assumed that older adults, living in urban areas and close to their families, have adequate access to health and community services, our experience has shown that this is not necessarily true. The older population, whether they live in rural or urban areas, are at risk for not receiving adequate medical care and necessary social services. This larger risk makes the elders vulnerable to many other medical and psychosocial complications. These include: (a) poor health, (b) nutritional deficits, (c) loneliness, (d) a lack of physical contact and mental stimulation, (e) disabilities, (f) spiritual distress, (g) depression, and (h) a relatively low quality of life.

Why do many of the elders fall under the category of a population at risk? They are a vulnerable population because of the progressive declining abilities that so often accompany aging and are part of chronic illness. Many older persons can no longer drive and thus lack transportation to health care facilities, shopping, and recreational activities. They may have communication difficulties because of poor hearing and vision; therefore, they avoid calling their doctors or others. Furthermore, because older persons often feel like a burden when they ask for help, they do not want to bother their children, or fear that if they ask too much too often, they will lose their independence. Many older persons and their families lack knowledge about what kinds of services are available in a community, or because they have limited or fixed incomes, are unable to make use of those services. Then, too, some have mobility problems and fear falling; therefore, they avoid going out on their own. Unless there is someone to shop for them or take them to appointments, they do without.

Most families do care. They visit, take the older parents to their homes for the holidays, take them shopping, out to dinner and to the movies, and sometimes to doctors' appointments. However, often families are out of touch with what is really going on medically and functionally with their older parents. Sometimes children don't want to face the reality of declining abilities in their parents. Some older parents hide their medical and functional problems from their children to protect them. Typically, it is not until a medical or other crisis occurs that an older parent and family members are forced to confront reality. Then, they may be uncertain about what course to take and turn to nurses and other helping professionals for assistance.

Health professionals, then, need theoretical frameworks that help them to identify situations that place elders at risk and that give direction for intervening to prevent or reduce the risks. The framework that we have chosen to work with in a community setting is the Corbin and Strauss Chronic Illness Trajectory Framework (henceforth referred to as the Trajectory Framework). We chose this framework because it is community oriented and directs attention to medical, functional, and related psychosocial problems that can make older adults vulnerable to a host of problems.

OVERVIEW OF CORBIN AND STRAUSS CHRONIC ILLNESS TRAJECTORY FRAMEWORK

The Trajectory Framework, as presented in Woog (1992), is a chronic illness management framework. It evolved out of years of research, both in homes and in hospitals (Corbin & Strauss, 1988; Fagerhaugh & Strauss, 1977; Strauss et al., 1984; Strauss, Fagerhaugh, Suczek, & Weiner, 1985; Strauss & Glaser, 1970; Strauss & Glaser, 1975). The value of the framework in working with an older group of persons living in the community is that:

1. It allows a flexible and inclusive approach to care. This is, it recognizes that older adults, like other adults, have a right to proper medical care and that their lives can be improved and prolonged as a result of that care.
2. It considers the older person and family central to the illness and disability management process; therefore, any decisions to be made regarding that management should be thoroughly discussed and negotiated by all parties, rather than imposed on the older parent by others.
3. Every effort is aimed at giving elders the resources and assistive devices they need to manage their own conditions at home for as long as possible.

4. It looks at the relationship among illness, functional ability, and social and psychological responses to illness and considers how these interact to create risks and how they can be manipulated to reduce risks.
5. It enables practitioners to look at illness and disability from a patient's perspective and to place emphasis on quality of life issues.

Definition of Terms

The term "trajectory" refers to a course of illness, including all the work and effort—by the ill person, family, and other professionals—that go into managing that course. Since chronic conditions are long term, over the course of chronic illness individuals often pass through two or more phases. The phases can be broken down into: (a) pretrajectory, (b) onset, (c) acute, (d) crisis, (e) stable, (f) unstable, (g) comeback, (h) downward, and (i) dying (see Table 3.1) (Corbin, 1995; Robinson et al., 1993). Persons can be in different phases of different illnesses, which can significantly complicate the medical management process.

The *pretrajectory* period is that which occurs before the onset of symptoms. If proper lifestyles and habits are maintained, some (but not all) chronic conditions can be prevented or at least the symptoms minimized. *Onset* denotes the beginning of symptoms and includes the diagnostic period and workup. *Stability* refers to the period when physical symptoms are more or less under control and the individual feels integrated and whole despite residual disability and loss. During the *acute* phase, a patient's illness and symptoms are serious enough to warrant hospitalization or skilled nursing care. *Comeback,* which follows an acute period or crisis, is the time devoted to the work of mending physically, regaining functional ability, reintegrating a shattered identity, and making social readjustments, all within the limitations imposed by the illness condition. In a *downward* phase, the objective is to slow the progress of disease by maintaining stable plateaus between each downward step and then making the social and psychological adjustments that are needed to adapt to lost roles and progressive symptoms. An *unstable* period is the time in an illness when symptoms may not be well controlled, complications develop, or psychosocial issues resurface, yet the individual is not so ill that hospitalization or skilled nursing care is required. In a *crisis,* life or identity is severely threatened, and immediate intervention is required to reduce the level of risk. *Dying* refers to the days and weeks before death, calling not only for physical comfort measures, but opportunities for persons to disengage from life and to make closure.

Other Concepts of the Framework

Other concepts important to this framework include: (a) the management team, (b) management processes, (c) context of management, and (d) interactive negotiative process.

Management Team

Because the task of managing chronic illness and aging extends beyond medical care and includes functional and psychosocial components, a multidisciplinary approach to management is called for (Bower, 1992; Swindle, Weyant, & Mar, 1994), whose efforts must be organized and coordinated. In a community setting, the task of organizing and coordinating services often falls on the nurse, the professional most likely to be going into the home to provide medical services.

Management Goals and Intervention Modes

The larger goals of management of chronic illness in older adults include: health promotion, prevention of illness complications, management of symptoms, handling of disabilities, and resolution of psychosocial issues. These goals can be reached through intervention modes that include, but are not limited to: case management, provision of direct care, patient advocacy, teaching, counseling, referrals, and making arrangements for resources.

Management Context

The context in which management will take place is important to consider when planning care. For example, knowing that an older cardiac patient lives in a house with stairs enables the nurse to assist the patient to organize activities of daily living in a manner that minimizes stair climbing. Assessing the patient includes obtaining information about the illness itself and its phasing, duration, symptoms, regimens, and complications. Additional contextual information necessary for planning care includes: the motivation of ill persons and their families to carry out regimens or to provide assistance; the older person's and family's psychosocial responses to illness; the availability of financial and others resources; and the nature of the home environment, that is, stairs to climb, location of bathrooms, proximity of neighbors, and so on (see Figure 3.1).

TABLE 3.1 Trajectory Phases

Phase	Definition	Goal of Management
Pretrajectory	Genetic factors or lifestyle behaviors that place an individual or community at risk for the development of a chronic condition.	Prevent onset of chronic illness.
Trajectory onset	Appearance of noticeable symptomes, includes period of diagnostic workup and announcement by biographical limbo as person begins to discover and cope with implications of diagnosis.	Form appropriate trajectory projection and scheme.
Stable	Illness course and symptoms are under control. Biography and everyday life activities are being managed within limitations of illness. Illness management centere in the home.	Maintain stability of illness, biography, and everyday life activities.
Unstable	Period of inability to keep symptoms under control or reactiviation of illness. Biographical disruption and difficulty in carrying out everyday life activities. Adjustments being made in regimen with care usually taking place at home.	Return to stable.
Acute	Severe and unrelieved symptoms or the development of illness complications necessitating hospitalization or bed rest to bring illness course under control. Biography and everyday life activities temporarily placed on hold or drastically cut back.	Bring illness under control and resume normal biography and everyday life activites.

TABLE 3.1 Trajectory Phases *(continued)*

Phase	Definition	Goal of Management
Crisis	Critical or life-threatening situation requiring emergency treatment or care. Biography and everyday life activities suspended until crisis passes.	Remove life threat.
Comeback	A gradual return to an acceptable way of life within limits imposed by disability or illness. Involves physical healing, limitations stretching through rehabilitative procedures, psychosocial coming to terms, and biographical reengagement with adjustments in everyday life activities.	Set in motion and keep going the trajectory projection and scheme.
Downward	Illness course characterized by rapid or gradual physical decline accompanied by increasing disability or difficulty in controlling symptoms. Requires biographical adjustment and alterations in everyday life activity with each major downward step.	To adapt to increasing disability with each major downward turn.
Dying	Final days or weeks before death. Characterized by gradual or rapid shutting down of body processes, biographical disengagement and closure, and relinquishment of everyday life interests and activities.	To bring closure, let go, and die peacefully.

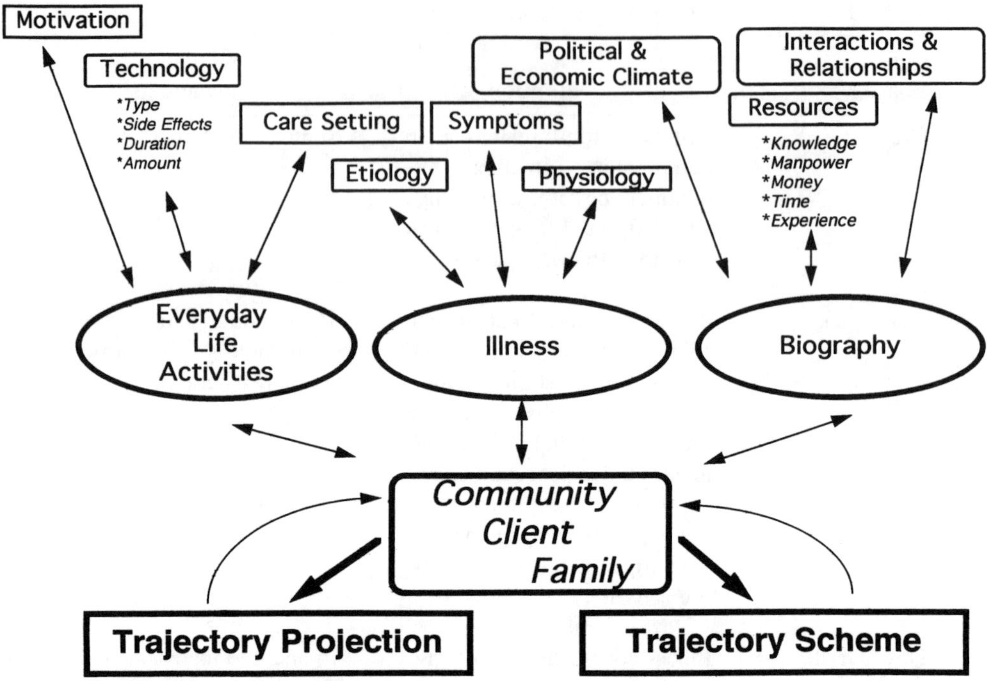

Figure 3.1 Context of Illness Management.

The health care management choices that are made have an impact on the course of a chronic illness and ultimately on the rate of aging and disability. In turn, psychosocial factors, such as the ability to come to terms with aging and illness and the availability of resources, affect health care choices. This interactive effect of illness, aging, and psychosocial factors is termed "reciprocal impact." It is out of this impact that many of the risk factors to which elders are vulnerable arise, as discussed in the previous section.

Interactive Negotiative Process

Giving older persons a voice in determining illness management and control over their futures is arrived at through a process termed the "interactive negotiative process" (see Figure 3.2).

This term indicates that the goals of care, as well as the means for their achievement, are the product of mutual discussion and agreement among

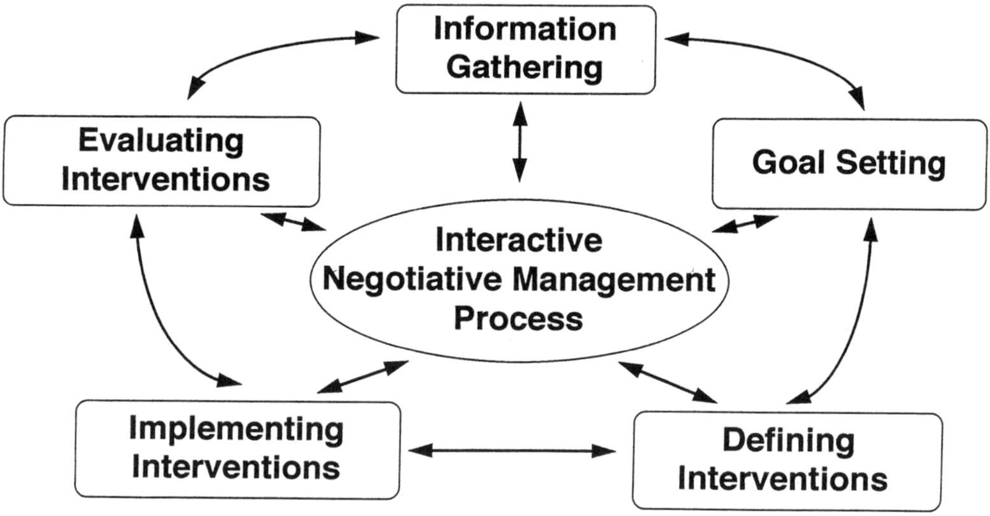

Figure 3.2 The Negotiative Management Process.

client, family, nurse, and other members of the management team. The relevant issue here is if the chronically ill person and family are not in agreement, or if the older person and family are not ready to make change or accept illness and disability, the plan, regardless of how great, will not be carried out fully. Health and allied professionals cannot—indeed, should not—make decisions for others. Since, ultimately the main responsibility for illness management falls upon the ill person and his or her family, their wishes should be respected. Older persons have the right to obtain a level of medical care that enables them to control their illness symtoms, minimize their disabilities, have some quality of life, and a peaceful death.

COMMUNITY-BASED MODELS OF CARE

Since most older persons reside in the community rather than in hospitals or long-term care facilities, and because they have difficulty reaching out for services for the reasons described previously, health care and other services must be brought to them. More and more, community-based programs are finding ways to bring services to elders or the elders to the services. One example of such a program is the On Lok Senior Health Services, which delivers comprehensive medical and support services to the frail elders. Their services are provided and managed by a multidisciplinary team (Cox, 1993). The On Lok model has been implemented in many cities in the United States through the Program of All-inclusive Care for the Elderly (PACE). Other examples of community-based models of care include: the Community Care Program in Illinois (Justice, 1988), the Bureau of Long-term Support in Wisconsin (Ball, 1989), the Family Caregivers Support Program in Pennsylvania (Pennsylvania Department on Aging, 1991), and the Seniors Agenda for Independent Living (SAIL) in Minnesota (Minnesota Department of Human Services, 1991). All of these programs attempt to overcome problems of access and fragmentation of services.

Nurse-Managed Centers

Nurses have traditionally reached out into the community to provide health care services to patients who otherwise might not have access. More recently, nurses have begun to value their unique contribution to patient care and well-being. These two aspects of nursing are fused in the concept of Nurse-Managed Centers (NMCs), which provide low-cost and patient-centered care in a community setting. Nurse-managed centers are innovative practice models that cost-effectively can meet the health care needs of many underserved populations in rural and urban settings (Mackey, Adams, & McNiel, 1994). NMCs have a long history dating back to 1893, with the Henry Street Settlement in New York City (Gorenberg & Cohen, 1994). NMCs may be located on site or offer off-site services. Off-site services are sometimes referred to as "centers without walls" (Walker, 1994).

Nurse-managed centers usually offer a range of services that differ from one center to the next depending on the needs of the target population and the clinical focus of the nurse providers. Predominantly, NMCs offer comprehensive health care services with an emphasis on health promotion, prevention, and illness management. NMCs offer opportunities for nurses to deliver autonomous, client-centered care using an interdisciplinary model (Walker, 1994). In addition, NMCs enable nurses to draw upon and utilize all of the theories, knowledge, and skills that they have acquired during their careers. Because nurses are directly accountable for the care they provide, they can take the time necessary to establish long-term therapeutic relationships, reach out and touch people in meaningful ways, and be responsive to the needs of the clients.

In NMCs, nurses have the freedom to make choices about the types of nursing care they will provide and explore the limits of care within the boundaries of their scope of practice. NMCs provide opportunities for teaching, case management, research, and for advanced practice (Doughty, 1989). Most of all, they enable nurses to manage the care of their clients: that is, to provide the broad-based holistic care that nurses are taught to provide but are so often restricted from giving because of institutional constraints.

APPLICATION OF THE TRAJECTORY FRAMEWORK IN A NURSE-MANAGED CENTER

Chai Health Center (CHC) is a community-based nurse-managed center that provides health care services to a population of older persons living in an urban setting. The health center is located in Chai House, a multiunit housing complex that has approximately 130 older residents, who range in age from 60 to 94. Since Chai House is an independent living facility, most residents are able to live on their own within this protected environment. Those with disabilities are required to receive assistance either from family members or hired help. As long as residents are able, through their own abilities or through the services of others, to care for themselves and not be a burden to the community, they may remain at Chai House. When residents can no longer meet their own living needs and the burden of care shifts to the community, they are no longer eligible to live there.

CHC is staffed by nursing faculty, undergraduate community-health nursing students, and graduate students whose focus is gerontological nursing. An interdisciplinary team approach to care is utilized. Nurses work collaboratively with

1. patients and their family members,
2. two social workers from the Jewish Family Service,
3. a retired pharmacist, and
4. two apartment-complex managers and other supportive staff such as dietary and maintenance.

Goals of Care at CHC

In keeping within the guidelines of the Trajectory Framework, the primary goals of care at CHC are:

1. to identify early those conditions that might place a resident at risk for medical and psychosocial problems and to contain those risks; and
2. to enhance elders' quality of life and enable them to live in their own homes for as long as possible.

Therefore, health care delivery in the NMC focuses on the following areas:

1. health promotion and disease prevention;
2. symptom management;
3. early detection of acute illness and prevention of chronic illness complications;
4. management of physical and mental disabilities;
5. preventing or minimizing psychosocial problems associated with aging and illness; and
6. locating and coordinating resources.

The means through which care is delivered include: direct physical care, teaching and demonstration, counseling and advising, advocating for clients, arrangement making, and referral making. A case management approach is used, and interventions are aimed at assisting residents to handle their disabilities, manage their illness conditions, while adjusting to the inevitable downward slope of their life course. Elders and their families are central to the management process, and decisions about care and placement are arrived at through negotiation among all parties.

CASE ILLUSTRATIONS

This section will illustrate, using case examples, how the Trajectory Framework has been used at CHC to guide care. The presentation will be organized around three foci of care: health promotion, prevention of complications, and handling of disabilities.

Health Promotion

It is in the pretrajectory phase of chronic illness that interventions focused on health promotion and disease prevention are most beneficial. In an effort to promote healthy lifestyles and prevent increasing chronicity and disability among our residents, a number of different projects have been undertaken. Educational classes are presented by the graduate and undergraduate nursing students every semester. Topics include classes on the value of diet and exercise in preventing osteoporosis, diabetes, and heart disease. The pharmacist also teaches classes with the students, which center on medications, their use and misuse, and some of the dangers and considerations when combining over-the-counter drugs with prescription medications. In addition to the classes, monthly bulletin boards are posted, emphasizing aspects of health and wellness that might be relevant to elders at any point in time. For example, in the summer the bulletin board might contain information on the dangers of sunburn and heatstroke and how to avoid these.

Each fall, at the requests of residents, the students run a flu clinic. Periodically, the nurses hold blood pressure, blood glucose, and hearing screening clinics. The hearing screenings are done by students from the Communication and Speech Disorders Department at San Jose State University. The nurses provide foot care to those elders who have vision problems or difficulties bending over. Exercise classes are held twice each week, and a do-it-yourself walking program is available to the residents. In addition, the social workers have "Loss and Grief" sessions with the elders and support group meetings for their adult children.

Prevention of Complications

It is through early detection and intervention that nurses can help prevent the complications that so often lead to acute problems or crises and subsequent destabilization of the illness course. An example comes from the case of Mrs. S.

> Mrs. S. is a 83-year-old woman with chronic hypertension and many residual disabilities from a stroke. A home visit was requested by Mr. S. because he said his wife "wasn't feeling very well." Mr. S. is the primary caregiver of his wife, although he recently accepted the assistance of a home health aide on a limited basis. After making the appropriate greetings, the nurse proceeded to do a thorough assessment of each area delineated in the Trajectory Framework. In doing so, the nurse discovered that Mrs. S. had 3+ edema of

both lower extremities, a blood pressure elevated above her usual range, and crackles in her lower lung bases. In addition, Mrs. S. admitted to being very depressed because she saw herself as deteriorating rapidly. She wondered how much longer she would be able to live at home. Another problem identified in the assessment was that Mrs. S. was not taking her Lasix as prescribed, because doing so resulted in urinary urgency and frequency. Her physical disabilities made it difficult for her to get to the bathroom on time, and so she was incontinent. If she tried to hurry, she increased her potential for falling.

This background information was part of the contextual conditions affecting the patient's management of her illness. The nurse and the couple agreed that the major problems were:

1. medical, the signs of early heart failure;
2. psychosocial, the depression and future living and illness course; and
3. functional, the inability to get to the bathroom on time.

With these problems in mind, the nurse and the couple proceeded to the next step, which was to define the goals of care. A long discussion ensued. Mr. S. wanted to increase the dosage of Lasix, without consulting the physician. Mrs. S. did not want to take even the basic dosage of Lasix, let alone an increased dosage. The conflict over which course of action to take provided the nurse with an opportunity to do health teaching about the illness, the medications, their handling, and their impact on the illness course. After listening to all the facts, Mrs. S. decided to take the medication. She did not want to develop severe heart failure, which might result in hospitalization. Mr. S. decided not to increase the medication dosage without checking with the physican. It was therefore agreed by the couple that they should call the physician and request an immediate appointment. The nurse counseled the couple on how to present the problem so that their request would be honored. The son was called to see if he would be available to drive his parents to the doctor.

The couple followed through and saw the physician. Mrs. S.'s Lasix was increased. To ease the contextual difficulty in getting to the bathroom on time, the nurse provided Mrs. S. with a portable commode from the CHC's store of equipment. With the additional medication, Mrs. S.'s condition stabilized. The complication was managed before it reached a critical point necessitating hospitalization. There still remained the problem of depression. An arrangement was made to have Mrs. S. meet with one of the social workers to discuss her feelings about loss of function, disability, and eventual death and dying.

Handling Disabilities

The handling of disabilities is an important task in any phase of chronic illness management. However, it is especially pertinent during the comeback, downward, and unstable phases. The next situation illustrates how the use of the Trajectory Framework and case management techniques enabled the staff to handle the disabilities of one of the residents.

> Mr. C. is an 80-year-old man with a long history of chronic, obstructive pulmonary disease. Over the past 5 years, his health has slowly declined with resulting functional disability. He could no longer walk without assistance, bathe himself, or clean his apartment. He was incontinent because of an uncontrolled prostate condition and stayed all day in his wet clothing. He did not clean up after his cat, so there was cat litter and food all over his apartment floor. When other residents started complaining to the apartment managers about Mr. C.'s condition, the managers requested a team conference. It was agreed that unless some changes were made in Mr. C.'s living arrangements, he could no longer reside at Chai House, because his ability to live independently was hampered.

Before attending the conference, each health care professional made a home visit to determine the extent and nature of the problems from their various perspectives. They talked to Mr. C. and his family members to learn their views on the situation. Finally, a group meeting was held with the following participants: the student nurse assigned to Mr. C.'s care, the nursing faculty, the registered nurse, a social worker from the Jewish Family Service, a social worker from Mr. C.'s doctor's office, one of the apartment managers, family members, and Mr. C. The meeting was held in Mr. C.'s apartment, where he would feel most comfortable. After each team member had an opportunity to express his or her concerns, the problems were prioritized. Mr. C. was given considerable voice in determining the goals of his care. Through negotiation, he was willing to accept the assistance of a home health aide because it would enable him to stay at Chai House, where he could have his beloved cat.

With the goal established, the next step was to develop a satisfactory plan for carrying out that goal. Mr. C. agreed to allow someone to help him bathe, clean his apartment, keep his medical appointments, and take his medications as prescribed. The family arranged to have a local pharmacy deliver the medications, consented to drive Mr. C. to medical appointments, and agreed to bear the financial costs of daily help. The social workers took on the tasks of helping Mr. C. and his family find acceptable help and alternative ways of paying for that help. The nurses provided Mr. C. with a walker and taught him how to use it. The nurses took on the responsibility of monitoring his health status between medical visits and giving him regular foot care, a hygienic area of major neglect. Ultimately, the nurses had the case management responsibility for overseeing, coordinating, and evaluating the effectiveness of care.

As a result of implementing the negotiated plan, Mr. C.'s medical condition stabilized. His living conditions improved, and he was able to remain at Chai House with his cat. Since Mr. C. is an older man who suffers from several chronic conditions, the staff know that another conference might be necessary in the future to help him manage the problems that will inevitably arise due to further downward changes in his multiple illness trajectories.

SUMMARY AND CONCLUSIONS

It is estimated that by the year 2030, almost 26 million older persons in the United States will be living alone. Of this population, approximately 9.7 million will have some health limitations (Zedlewski & McBride, 1992). These staggering figures clearly indicate the need for planning ahead and implementing models of health care delivery to meet future demands. Without such changes, the present health care delivery system will be overwhelmed.

What kind of system is needed? Obviously, one that meets the health care challenges and needs of populations most at risk for inadequate health care and the problems that result. One such population is older adults, who not only have a high incidence of chronic illness, but because of their age, immobility, and other limitations, are very much at risk for not having their medical conditions adequately managed. Long-term rather than short-term solutions are needed to solve this problem.

Solutions are difficult to find because hospital costs are rising and insurers are gaining increased control over how health care is delivered. While nurses might not be able to change these facts, they can devise methods of delivering quality care that fit within that structure, in particular: low-cost, long-term, community-based care that is chronic illness focused.

Neigborhood-run, nurse-managed centers, such as the one described in this chapter, can fill many of the health care delivery gaps that put our aging population at risk. Nurse practitioners and nursing students can deliver low-cost, holistic, community-based primary care to older populations in a variety of settings including NMCs. By utilizing theoretical frameworks that focus on the specific problems of chronic illness and aging, nurses can identify potential situations of risk and intervene early to prevent or minimize the problems.

However, given the present social climate, legislators are reluctant to commit more funds to medical and social programs for any group of persons. Before community-based care programs for elders can be expanded to meet present and future needs, the cost-effectiveness of NMCs and other programs must be documented through research (Greene, Lovely, & Ondrich, 1993; Hansen, Spedtsberg, & Schroll, 1992; Rossum et al., 1993; Scott & Moneyham, 1995).

It is a troubling but exciting time in health care. As the traditional ways of health care delivery disintegrate, the opportunity exists to develop new systems that are forward looking. Nurses must take the lead and reach out into communities both rural and urban to work with populations at risk. NMCs are an innovative prototype of health care delivery that fit with both the health care needs of specific populations and the existing social climate. NMCs along with theoretical frameworks that address today's health care issues, namely chronic illness, can create powerful forces that shape the future while reducing risks and enhancing quality of life in older adults.

REFERENCES

Ball, C. (1989). *Long-term care management: A policy analysis of four exemplary models.* Public Policy Institute, American Association of Retired Persons [AARP]. Washington, DC: AARP.

Bower, K. A. (1992). *Case management by nurses.* Washington, DC: American Nurses Publishing.

Charmaz, K. (1983). Loss of self: Fundamental form of suffering in the chronically ill. *Sociology of Health & Illness, 5*(4), 168–195.

Colley, C. A., & Lucas, L. M. (1993). Polypharmacy: The cure becomes the disease. *Journal of General Internal Medicine, 8,* 278–284.

Corbin, J. (1995). Chronic illness as a general phenomenon. In S. Smeltzer & B. Bare (Eds.), *Brunner and Suddarth's textbook of medical-surgical nursing* (pp. 317–324). Philadelphia: J. B. Lippincott.

Corbin, J., & Strauss, A. (1988). *Unending work and care.* San Francisco: Jossey-Bass.

Corbin, J., & Strauss, A. (1991). A nursing model for chronic illness management based upon the trajectory framework. *Scholarly Inquiry for Nursing Practice, 5*(3), 155–174.

Cox, C. (1993). *The frail elderly: Problems, needs, and community responses.* Westport, CT: Auburn House.

Doughty, S. E. D. (1989). The CNS in a nurse-managed center. In A. B. Hamric & J. A. Spross (Eds.), *The clinical nurse specialist in theory and practice* (pp. 415–434). Philadelphia: W. B. Saunders.

Fagerhaugh, S. Y., & Strauss, A. L. (1977). *Politics of pain management: Staff-patient interaction.* Menlo Park, CA: Addison-Wesley.

Gambert, S. R., Grossberg, G. T., & Morley, J. E. (1994). How many drugs does your aged patient need? *Patient Care,* March 30, 61–72.

Gorenberg, B., & Cohen, J. (1994). Nurse-managed centers: An innovative structure for nursing education and care. *International Nursing Review, 41*(5), 148–150.

Greene, V. L., Lovely, M. E., & Ondrich, J. I. (1993). The cost-effectiveness of community services in a frail elderly population. *Gerontologist, 33*(2), 177–189.

Guralnik, J. M., LaCroix, A. Z., Everett, D. F., & Kovar, M. G. (1989, May 26). *Aging in the eighties: The prevalence of comorbidity and its association with disability* (advance data from Vital and Health Statistics of the National Center for Health Statistics, No. 170). Washington, DC: U.S. Department of Health and Human Services, Public Health Service, Centers for Disease Control.

Hansen, F. R., Spedtsberg, K., & Schroll, M. (1992). Geriatric follow-up by home visits after discharge from hospital: A randomized controlled trial. *Age and Ageing, 21,* 445–450.

Justice, D. (1988). *State long-term care reform: Development of community care systems in six states.* Washington, DC: National Governors Association.

Kane, R., Ouslander, J., & Abrass, I. (1994). *Essentials of clinical geriatrics.* New York: McGraw Hill, Health Professions Division.

Mackey, T. A., Adams, J., & McNiel, N. O. (1994). Nursing centers: Service as a business. *Journal of Nurse Economics, 12*(5), 276–279.

Minnesota Department of Human Services. (1991). *A strategy for long-term care in the state of Minnesota, developed in response to the SAIL report.* St. Paul, MN: Department of Human Services.

National Center for Health Statistics. (1992). *Current estimates from the National Health Interview Survey, 1991* (Series 10, No. 184). U.S. Department of Health and Human Services.

Pennsylvania Department of Aging. (1991). *Family caregiver support program: Final evaluation report.* Harrisburg, PA: Pennsylvania Department on Aging.

Robinson, C. A. (1993). Managing life with a chronic condition: The story of normalization. *Qualitative Health Research, 3*(1), 6–28.

Robinson, L., Bevil, C., Arcangelo, V., Reifsnyder, J., Rothman, N., & Smeltzer, S. (1993). Operationalizing the Corbin & Strauss trajectory model for elderly clients with chronic illness. *Scholarly Inquiry for Nursing Practice, 7*(4), 253–268.

Rossum, E. van, Frederiks, C. M. A., Philipsen, H., Portengen, K., Wiskerke, J., & Knipschild, P. (1993). Effects of preventive home visits to elderly people. *British Medical Journal, 307,* 27–32.

Scott, C. B., & Moneyham, L. (1995). Perceptions of senior residents about a community-based nursing center. *Image: Journal of Nursing Scholarship, 27*(3), 181–186.

Strauss, A., & Corbin, J. (1988). *Shaping a new health care system.* San Francisco: Jossey-Bass.

Strauss, A., Corbin, J., Fagerhaugh, S., Glaser, B., Maines, D., Suczek, B., & Weiner, C. (1984). *Chronic illness and the quality of life* (2nd ed.). St. Louis: Mosby.

Strauss, A., Fagerhaugh, S., Suczek, B., Weiner, C. (1985). *Social organization of medical work.* Chicago: University of Chicago Press.

Strauss, A., & Glaser, B. (1970). *Anguish: A case history of a dying trajectory.* Mill Valley, CA: Sociology Press.

Strauss, A., & Glaser, B. (1975). *Chronic illness and the quality of life* (1st ed.). St. Louis: Mosby.

Swindle, D. N., Weyant, J. L., & Mar, P. S. (1994). Nurse case management: Collaborative beyond the hospital walls. *Journal of Case Management, 3*(2), 51–55.

Walker, P. H. (1994). Dollars and sense in health reform: Interdisciplinary practice and community nursing centers. *Nursing Administrative Quarterly, 19*(1), 1–11.

Woog, P. (Ed.). (1992). *The chronic illness trajectory framework: The Corbin and Strauss nursing model.* New York: Springer.

Zedlewski, S. R., & McBride, T. D. (1992). The changing profile of the elderly: Effects on future long-term care needs and financing. *Milbank Quarterly, 70*(2), 247–275.

CHAPTER 4

Chronic Pain in the Elderly

Keela A. Herr and Paula R. Mobily

Pain is the most poorly managed in those most defenseless against it—the young and the elderly.

—Liebeskind & Melzack, 1987

Pain is a significant problem for many elderly persons. Because of the high incidence of chronic diseases, falls, and other health problems associated with aging, elders are at increased risk for experiencing both acute and chronic pain. Although there have been tremendous advances in the scientific understanding and clinical management of pain, the special needs and considerations of elders with pain is a neglected area. As the 21st century approaches, elders will increase in both number and proportion of the population, thus increasing the importance of the problem of pain to society. Relatively little information exists concerning the prevalence and impact of pain and the current status of pharmacologic and nonpharmacologic management of pain in this population. The Agency for Health Care Policy and Research (AHCPR) has devoted significant resources to development of guidelines that provide recommendations for pain management in acute postoperative pain and cancer pain (Acute Pain Management Guideline Panel, 1992; Jacox, Carr, Payne, et al., 1994). Both guidelines substantiate the lack of research to direct the approach to care of the elderly patient with pain.

Although older adults certainly can experience both acute and chronic pain, they are at greater risk for pathological disorders that result in chronic pain, including musculoskeletal diseases, diabetic neuropathies, atherosclerotic peripheral vascular disease, cancer, trigeminal neuralgia, and herpes zoster among others (Davis, 1988; Foley, 1985; Gordon, 1979). Chronic pain often is more complex, requires multidimensional management strategies, and is more often neglected by health professionals (Closs, 1994). Also, chronic pain in older adults may result in different outcomes and require different treatment strategies than young or middle-aged individuals. These issues, coupled with known misconceptions or misbeliefs concerning pain in elders, create barriers to quality care of those elders with pain. Attention to these issues is critical in promoting optimal pain management for this population and should capture the attention of those interested in promoting improved pain management for elders.

It is not the intent of the authors to provide a manual of care for the elder patient in pain. The purpose of this chapter is to examine the key issues related to pain assessment and management in this population and to make recommendations for practice and research. The emphasis is on chronic pain, although most of the issues relate to both acute and chronic pain conditions.

Prevalence of Pain in Older Adults

It is difficult to estimate accurately the general frequency of pain problems for elders because of the lack of systematic epidemiological investigation (Butler & Gastel, 1980; B. A. Ferrell & B. R. Ferrell, 1991; Harkins, 1988; Harkins, Kwentus, & Price, 1984; Melding, 1991; Portenoy & Farkash, 1988). Most of the available information about prevalence of pain in this population is limited to specific body parts or based on symptoms reported to physicians or pain clinics and information obtained during hospitalization or long-term care institutionalization. Data from these sources are not representative of the prevalence of pain in the general older population.

Although limited, available data suggest that approximately 36%–83% of the elderly population report some degree of pain that may interfere with life's activities and quality of life (Brody & Kleban, 1983; Demlow, Liang, & Eaton, 1986; B. A. Ferrell, B. R. Ferrell, & Osterweil, 1990; Mobily, Herr, Clark, & Wallace, 1994; Moss, Lawton, & Glicksman, 1991; Rousseau & Calvin, 1993; Roy & Thomas, 1986, 1987; Thomas & Roy, 1988). Population-based studies estimate that 25%–50% of community-dwelling older adults suffer as a result of chronic pain problems (Brattberg, Mats, & Anders, 1989; Crook, Rideout, & Browne, 1984). Among nursing home residents, the prevalence of pain appears to be even higher, with estimates that 49%–83% of nursing home residents experience chronic pain (B. A. Ferrell, B. R. Ferrell, et al., 1990; Lau-Ting & Phoon, 1988; Roy & Thomas, 1986).

The significant percentage of elders experiencing pain in their lives mandates that researchers and practitioners make a commitment to addessing the needs for optimal pain management within this population.

IMPACT OF PAIN ON THE QUALITY OF LIFE

Because chronicity is a key characteristic of pain in this population, the concept of quality of life is of major importance, and improving quality of life becomes a key outcome of intervention. B. R. Ferrell, Wisdom, and Wenzel (1989) and B. R. Ferrell, Grant, Padilla, Vemuri, and Rhiner (1991) have proposed a model useful for understanding the interface of pain and quality of life that incorporates a physical dimension, involving symptoms and activity; a psychological dimension, including anxiety and depression; a social dimension, involving caregiver burden, roles, and relationships; and a spiritual dimension of pain incorporating suffering and the meaning of pain to the individual. As this model illustrates, chronic pain can impact a wide range of activities, resulting in disability and severe lifestyle changes. General quality of life correlates of pain in older adults include impaired functional abilities, sleep disturbances, altered nutrition, fatigue, impaired cognitive functioning, mood alterations, including anxiety and depression, and impaired or diminished social and recreational activities (Brody & Kleban, 1983; B. R. Ferrell et al., 1989; B. R. Ferrell, Wisdom, Wenzel, & Brown, 1990; Guccione, Meenan, & Anderson, 1989; Herr, Mobily, Wallace, & Chung, 1991; Lavsky-Shulan et al., 1985; Liang et al., 1984; Mobily et al., 1994; Parmalee, Smith, & Katz, 1993).

Quality of life variables are critically important in measuring the impact of chronic pain and provide important outcome measures of successful intervention. Although the research cited previously provides an important beginning base of data for understanding the impact of pain on quality of life, systematic research is needed to understand better the physical, psychological, social, and spiritual impact of pain on this population and the intervariable relationships that moderate the phenomenon.

Pain and Mood/Depression

Although the impact of chronic pain on mood/depression was acknowledged previously, the importance of this relationship warrants additional discussion. Chronic pain is likely to be a cause of depression, but it is often viewed as a symptom of depression producing similar behaviors. Although estimates of depression in chronic pain populations have varied widely, the majority of studies report the coexistence of depression in a significant proportion of chronic pain patients (Blumer & Heilbronn, 1981; Kerns & Turk, 1984; Kleinke & Spangler, 1988; Romano & Turner, 1985).

Not only are elders more susceptible to chronic pain and pain-producing illnesses, but they are at considerable risk for depressive disorders independent of pain (Blazer, Hughes, & George, 1987; Harkins et al., 1984; Parmalee, Katz, & Lawton, 1991). Analysis of the prevalence of this association for elders has been limited; however, several studies have provided empirical documentation of the link between depression and pain in this population (Herr, Mobily, & Smith, 1993; Magni, Schifano, & DeLeo, 1985; Moss et al., 1991; Parmalee et al., 1991; Sorkin, Rudy, Hanlon, Turk, & Stieg, 1990; Williamson & Schulz, 1992).

Positive relationships among depression and pain-related variables, particularly pain intensity, have been documented (Brown, Nicassio, & Wallston, 1989; Doan & Wadden, 1989; Haythornthwaite, Seiber, & Kerns, 1991; Herr et al., 1993; Keefe, Wilkins, Cook, Crisson, & Muhlbaier, 1986; Parmalee et al., 1991). Also, the relationship among pain, depression, and functioning has been verified empirically. Depressed chronic pain patients consistently report lower levels of functioning and greater interference in a variety of common daily activities than those not depressed (Brown et al., 1989; Doan & Wadden, 1989; Haley, Turner, & Romano, 1985; Haythornthwaite et al., 1991; Herr & Mobily, 1992; Herr et al., 1993; Keefe et al., 1986).

Functional disability has been shown to mediate the relationship between pain and depressed affect in elders (Williamson & Schulz, 1992). Additionally, in the general population, the impact of pain on social, recreational, family, and occupational activities, as well as perceived control over life, significantly affects the relationship between pain and depression (Rudy, Kerns, & Turk, 1988), and this relationship seems to be more pronounced in elders (Turk, Okifuji, & Scharff, 1994). The availability of social support has also been shown to play an important role in depression among elderly chronic pain patients (Turk, Kerns, & Rosenberg, 1992). These studies, though limited in number, emphasize the importance of carefully assessing the impact of pain on functional activities and the availability of social support when working with the elderly client. Further research in this area is warranted.

KEY ISSUES RELATED TO OPTIMAL PAIN MANAGEMENT IN OLDER ADULTS

Inadequate Knowledge

One of the major barriers to effective pain management in all age groups is inadequate knowledge on the part of health care professionals, significant others, and the patient. Although knowledge and strategies in pain management have evolved substantially, medical and nursing knowledge and clinical practice have not followed suit (Diekmann & Wassem, 1991; McCaffery, Ferrell, O'Neil-Page, Lester, & Ferrell, 1990).

Research has identified some of the reasons for poor pain management with the general population, including deficiencies in the educational system regarding pain control (Diekmann & Wassem, 1991; B. R. Ferrell, McGuire, & Donovan, 1993; Graffam, 1990; McCaffery & Ferrell, 1992; Watt-Watson & Watson, 1989); incorrect information in textbooks (B. R. Ferrell, McCaffery, & Rhiner, 1992); lack of knowledge related to pain assessment and management by health professionals, including practitioners, faculty, and students (Brunier, Carson, & Harrison, 1995; Dalton, Diekmann & Wassem, 1991; Marks & Sachar, 1973; Wallace, Reed, Pasero, & Olsson, 1995); and lack of clinical skills to assess and manage pain by physicians and nurses (Bonica, 1990; Dalton, 1989; Rankin & Snider, 1984; Sheidler, McGuire, Grossman, & Gilbert, 1992; Teske, Daut, & Cleeland, 1983).

To date, there has been little research to identify the factors specifically affecting the management of pain in elders; however, considering the inaccuracies and inadequacies of the knowledge base for pain management of the general population, one can expect that even greater deficiencies might exist concerning the older population. In fact, B. R. Ferrell and B. A. Ferrell (1992) found that surprisingly little attention has been focused on the management of pain in geriatrics. Of 11 leading textbooks of geriatric medicine, only 2 devoted chapters to the approach and management of pain. Similarly, a review of eight geriatric nursing textbooks revealed less than 18 pages, from more than 5,000 total pages of text, devoted to pain. Of the over 4,000 papers on pain published annually, less than 1% focus on pain in elders (Melding, 1991). Given this lack of attention to content that addresses specific concerns and strategies related to managing pain in elders, the inaccuracies in the knowledge base of those caring for elders is not surprising, but of significant concern. The Task Force for Pain in the

Elderly from the International Association for the Study of Pain (IASP) has developed model curricula for health professionals that include essential content on pain management for this population. Use of an established curriculum in professional health education would alleviate many of the problems noted in this section.

General Misconceptions

Misbeliefs are all too common in the minds of practitioners, educators, students, and, subsequently, for significant others and the elders themselves. In part, these unsubstantiated beliefs are related to the limited research base concerning pain in this population. The most significant of these will be discussed in the following sections on assessment and pharmacologic and nonpharmacologic management of pain. However, two general misconceptions need to be addressed that affect the quality of pain management in elders in a global sense.

One of the major misconceptions regarding pain in elders is the belief that pain is simply an expected and natural outcome of growing old (Butler & Gastel, 1980; Melding, 1991; Witte, 1989). This pain-related ageism leads to lack of aggressive assessment and intervention for pain conditions affecting elders. In fact, pain is not an inevitable part of aging, and its presence necessitates assessment, diagnosis, and treatment as in any age group.

A second misconception is the belief by some that pain sensitivity or perception decreases with age (Enck, 1991). Results of experimental studies on pain perception in elders fail to report, conclusively, age-related differences in pain perception (Harkins & Chapman, 1976, 1977; Harkins et al., 1984; Harkins, Price, & Martelli, 1986; Tucker, Andrew, Ogle, & Davison, 1989). In fact, in a review of studies published between 1940 and 1990 (B. A. Ferrell, 1991), three demonstrated an increase in pain threshold in this population, one demonstrated a modification of the threshold, and five studies demonstrated no change in threshold. Although elders may be slower to perceive or respond to pain, the research does not support that they feel pain less intensely. There are instances of atypical presentations of clinical pain, including silent MIs and the absence of abdominal pain in elders with peptic ulcer disease (Bender, 1989); however, these reports cannot be generalized to all disorders that result in pain or to all elders who experience MIs or ulcers. Without convincing empirical evidence demonstrating the accuracy of this belief, it must not be assumed that elders experience less pain than younger adults. The unfortunate consequence of stereotyping elders as experiencing less pain undoubtedly results in needless suffering and decreased quality of life for this population.

ASSESSMENT OF CHRONIC PAIN IN OLDER ADULTS

Inadequate assessment of pain and pain-related outcomes is an important barrier to optimal pain management irrespective of age or type of pain. Both the implementation and evaluation of interventions in the care of elders and the evaluation of treatments in controlled studies require accurate assessment of clinical pain. Not surprisingly, researchers have found that pain in elders is often poorly assessed (Dalton, 1989; Faherty & Grier, 1984; Ferrell, Ferrell, et al., 1990; Rankin & Snider, 1984; Teske, Daut, & Cleeland, 1983). Discussion of some of the major issues related to assessment of pain in elders follows.

Misconceptions Related to Pain Assessment

If the elder does not complain of pain, he or she must not have pain. This unfortunate misconception often leads to poor pain assessment and ineffective pain control. Failure to report pain must not be interpreted as absence of pain. Beliefs that interfere with report of pain include age-related stoicism; belief that pain is an inevitable part of aging, or that nothing can be done to relieve it (Ferrell, Ferrell, et al., 1990; Foley, 1985; McCaffery & Beebe, 1989; Melding, 1991); fear that pain may be indicative of more severe pathology or even impending death; and fear of the consequences of acknowledging pain such as the need for hospitalization, diagnostic tests, additional expenses, or loss of independence and autonomy (Copp, 1990; Hofland, 1992; Portenoy, 1988). Additionally, many elders accept the role of "passive recipient" of health care and assume that physicians and nurses know when they hurt (Hickey, 1988) and, if there were something that could be done to relieve their pain, it would be prescribed or initiated. Finally, Ferrell, Ferrell, et al. found that many elders in long-term care facilities fail to report pain and request pain management strategies because they do not want to be a bother to the staff or, more disturbingly, because they get tired of asking staff for help with pain management.

Unfortunately, many health professionals assume that older clients who are cognitively intact can accurately and succinctly describe their pain;

however, with elder clients in particular, the terminology used to indicate pain may not communicate accurately the extent of the individual's discomfort. For example, to elder clients, an "ache," "soreness," or "hurt" may represent a level of discomfort necessitating treatment that may be dismissed as inconsequential by the health professional.

Measurement of Pain and Pain-Related Constructs

Although research has been conducted on pain assessment in other age groups, there has been little systematic investigation of pain assessment in elders. In 1992, the Acute Pain Management Guideline Panel concluded that traditional measurement instruments for pain assessment lack established psychometric properties specific to elders. The limited empirical support for use of standardized assessment tools in elders makes it more difficult for practitioners to be knowledgeable and confident about the best approach to assessment. Research is needed to delineate the instruments that work most effectively with elders and to identify factors that can assist the practitioner in selecting an appropriate instrument. In addition to individual scales that quickly evaluate the sensory intensity of pain (e.g., visual analog scale (VAS), verbal descriptor scale, and numeric rating scale), multidimensional measures have been developed and should be used if assessment of pain is to be comprehensive. The ultimate common goal is to represent the pain experience accurately, which necessitates development and use of reliable, valid, and comprehensive measures.

Because pain intensity is one of the key components of pain assessment, it often is used as a benchmark for comparison of pain conditions over time and to determine the effectiveness of intervention strategies. However, research supporting the use of selected pain intensity measures with elders is limited. While no single pain measure is adequate for all elders or for all types of pain, there are several rating scales available that are appropriate for use with elders. Although prior research suggests that elders may have difficulty using the VAS (Jensen, Karoly, & Braver, 1986; Kremer, Atkinson, & Ignelzi, 1981), there is a void of focused investigations examining factors that influence the ability of elders to use it successfully. Other tools such as numeric rating scales and verbal numeric rating scales may serve this population better than the more abstract VAS, although in a study examining the use of five pain intensity measures within an elderly sample, Herr and Mobily (1991) found that elders were able to use the VAS successfully.

Some pain assessment scales that have been tested with specific populations, such as facial scales developed for assessment of pain intensity with children, might be appropriate for use in elders. Most have preliminary psychometric evaluation that supports their use; however, further study is needed (Beyer & Aradine, 1986; Bieri, Reeve, Champion, Addicoat, & Ziegler, 1990; McGrath, DeVeber, & Hearn, 1985; Tyler, Tu, Douthit, & Chapman, 1993).

The utility or usability and preference for a given tool are issues that are not often addressed, but certainly are relevant when determining interest in and use of a selected tool. Verbal descriptor scales appear to be easy for elders to use and are often preferred (Herr & Mobily, 1991). Additional testing of the reliability, validity, and utility of the VAS and related measures with elders is needed, as well as testing of elders with varying educational backgrounds.

Identifying tools that address the specific components involved in the elder's overall functioning is important. In addition to providing a comprehensive assessment of pain and its impact, the use of these scales is particularly important to monitor change over time and to document the effect of interventions.

With improving the quality of life as a key goal in management of chronic pain in elders, it is crucial that the assessment encompass more than an evaluation of the pain intensity. Unfortunately, nurses often fail to gather data about the effect of pain on the quality of life (Dalton, 1989). Numerous instruments have been developed and tested for use with elders that can provide a comprehensive evaluation of several quality of life domains related specifically to pain. The West Haven-Yale Multidimensional Pain Inventory (Kerns, Turk, & Rudy, 1985) and the Pain Disability Index (Tait, Pollard, Margolis, Duckro, & Krause, 1987) are useful instruments with established psychometric data from older adults that address the overall impact of pain on domains related to the quality of life. Clinical experience with these tools has revealed that the majority of cognitively intact older adults have little difficulty with the use of these instruments, although modifications in the size of presentation of the scales used, as well as careful and sometimes repeated instructions by the clinician or investigator, often simplifies its use and ensures greater reliability of the data collected.

Because of the significance of the relationship between pain and depression, assessment of the presence or absence of depression is important. Chronic pain alone can cause significant impairment; however, the interaction between pain and depression mandates careful assessment to determine if there is coexistence of these clinical problems. The presence of dysphoria or depression can be evaluated through the use of several scales, including the Geriatric Depression Scale (Yesavage et al., 1983), the Beck Depression Inventory (Beck, Ward, Mendelson, Mock, & Erbaugh, 1961), and the Center for Epidemiologic Studies Depression Scale, or CES-D (Radloff, 1977), among others.

Older people with chronic pain have been found to have more adaptive pain coping beliefs than younger people (Kotler-Cope & Gerber, 1993), which may impact the severity of pain reported and the impact pain is having on their lives. Gathering information on coping status and coping factors is important to plan appropriate interventions (Walker, Akinsanya, Davis, & Marcer, 1990), but often is omitted when nurses assess pain problems (Dalton, 1989). The Coping Strategies Questionnaire, or CSQ (Rosenstiel & Keefe, 1983), is an instrument designed to assess quantitatively coping strategies for the individual experiencing pain. In addition to identifying patterns of coping, the tool also includes two measures of the perceived effectiveness of coping strategies that can provide valuable information for pain management.

Complete assessment should elicit information about functional health as well. Instruments targeting specific functional domains are available and include the Katz ADL Scale (Katz, Ford, Moskowitz, Jackson, & Jaffe, 1963), the Instrumental Activities of Daily Living Scale (Lawton & Brody, 1969), and the Barthel Index (Mahoney & Barthel, 1965), among others.

Factors Affecting Assessment

Because some elders experience cognitive, sensory-perceptual, and psychomotor changes that might interfere with their ability to conceptualize the pain measure and respond appropriately, it is essential that these factors be considered as possible confounding variables in the ability to respond correctly to the various assessment measures. Adaptations can be made to accommodate many of these impairments. Although discussion of these impairments is beyond the scope of this chapter, they are discussed in some detail in a previous publication by the authors (Herr & Mobily, 1991).

Cognitive impairment, however, is a more challenging impairment that presents serious barriers to the assessment of pain in elders. Cognitive deficits may lead to underreporting of pain due to problems in recalling, interpreting, or communicating pain symptoms or to exaggeration or fabrication of pain complaints (Parmalee et al., 1993).

Cognitive impairment is an age-related phenomenon, increasingly prevalent after the age of 65. Dementia, the most common form of cognitive impairment in elders, may cause decrease or loss of memory, intelligence, thinking ability, calculation, problem-solving, judgment, comprehension, recognition, orientation, attention, and visuospatial skills (Dastoor, Schwartz, & Kurzman, 1991)—skills crucial to the successful use of instruments to measure various aspects of pain and necessitating adjustments in the assessment process.

Many practical mental status tests appropriate for use with elders are available. The most notable include the Cognitive Capacity Screening Examination (CCSE) (Jacobs, Bernhard, Delgado, & Strain, 1977), the Short Portable Mental Status Questionnaire (Pfeiffer, 1975), and the Mini-Mental State Examination (Folstein, Folstein, & McHugh, 1975). Because studies have suggested that current cognitive screening procedures may require a certain level of education for the accurate measurement of cognitive impairment, caution must be taken with populations that are nonliterate or semiliterate. The clock drawing procedure is a method of evaluating cognitive impairment that is relatively free from cultural and educational bias and has been used successfully to identify cognitive and visuospatial impairment in elderly subjects (Dastoor et al., 1991; Shulman, Shedletsky, & Silver, 1986; Wolf-Klein, Silverstone, Levy, Brod, & Breuer, 1989).

Basic assessment parameters for the cognitively impaired elder can be suggested, but serve merely as guides because of the very limited empirical support to date. For the older adults with minimal to mild cognitive impairment, soliciting their perceptions should be a primary focus of assessment, and efforts should be made to obtain self-reports before assuming it is not possible. Parmalee et al. (1993), studying 758 patients in nursing homes, concluded that although cognitively impaired elders may slightly underreport experienced pain, their self-reports were as valid as those of cognitively intact individuals. With the cognitively impaired older adults, incorporation of the family and significant other into the evaluation process is useful in making judgments regarding their pain experience. Recognition of pathologies and procedures known to cause pain also can help identify the presence of discomfort.

When the level of cognitive impairment interferes with self-report, evaluation of verbal and nonverbal behaviors is the approach used most often to assess pain. Observation of pain behavior has been more successful with various kinds of chronic pain than acute pain, but is limited by the fact that pain behaviors are highly specific to particular pain syndromes (Chapman & Syrjala, 1990). Marzinski (1991) examined the assessment strategies of nurses in long-term care facilities (LTCF) and found that staff based their assessment of pain on deviations from normal behavior patterns. The greater problem arises when the patient is already cognitively impaired on presentation and there is no baseline data for reference. Do vocalizations indicate pain? Are there any changes in behavior that the family perceives as indicative of discomfort? Are some of the body movements exhibited pain related rather than disease related? What changes in daily activities, gait, rest pattern, social interactions, and common routines are evident that might reflect discomfort?

To date, there are no clear, reliably sensitive behavioral indicators of pain in cognitively impaired older adults. Although Hurley, Volicer, Hanrahan, Houde, and Volicer (1992) developed a scale to assess discomfort in noncommunicative patients with advanced Alzheimer's Disease, this scale is representative of a number of "discomfort" states, including fever and nausea, and not a clear reflection of pain. An assessment strategy that might be useful for assessing cognitively impaired elderly is the use of facial expression analysis. Researchers have identified facial expressions that convey information about pain (Craig, Hyde, & Patrick, 1991; Prkachin, 1992) that appear to be common to a variety of pain states; however, there is no evidence that these expression characteristics are universal indicators of pain.

The complexities of conducting research with this population is most likely a major reason this population has been neglected by researchers, but the need for further study to direct practice with the cognitively impaired is critical. Until empirical support is available, practitioners must, nonetheless, proceed with interactions with patients and significant others to gather the best data possible on which to make judgments about pain and its management.

MANAGEMENT AND INTERVENTION STRATEGIES

There is growing recognition that older adults can benefit tremendously from more aggressive management of the chronic pain they experience, particularly when treatment approaches are used that are multimodal, combining both pharmacologic and nonpharmacologic modalities. Indeed, a multimodal approach using pharmacologic and nonpharmacologic strategies often is more effective (Butler & Gastel, 1980; B. A. Ferrell & B. R. Ferrell, 1991; Haley & Dolce, 1986; Harkins et al., 1984; Jay & Miller, 1990; Portenoy & Farkash, 1988; Roy & Thomas, 1986; Tait, 1993).

The Gate Control Theory, formulated and later modified by Melzack and Wall (1965, 1982), provides a powerful theoretical basis for multimodal management of pain. Pain is recognized as a complex, multidimensional experience interrelating three components: (1) the sensory discriminative (physical); (2) the affective-motivational (psychological); and (3) the cognitive-interpretative (cognitive) aspects of an individual's perception. A gating mechanism in the dorsal horn of the spinal column allows pain to be reduced or modulated at four points: (1) the peripheral site of pain; (2) in the spinal cord itself; (3) in the brain stem; and (4) in the cerebral cortex. Nonnarcotic analgesics, application of heat and cold, and local anesthetics alter the release of nociceptive substances and decrease accompanying muscle spasm at the peripheral site of pain. In the spinal cord, application of heat and cold, massage, and direct electrical stimulation awaken large nerve fibers and interfere with transmission of pain impulses. Electrical stimulation, acupuncture, and administration of narcotic analgesics can reduce effectively or eliminate transmission of pain impulses in the brain stem. Finally, cognitive-behavioral techniques such as relaxation, imagery, distraction, music therapy, hypnosis, and cognitive therapy, as well as administration of narcotic and narcotic antagonist analgesics work primarily through action in the cerebral cortex (Donovan, 1989). Use of a combination of interventions that exert their effects at different levels of the peripheral and central nervous system will result in more effective management of pain.

Research examining the effects of age on various pain control modalities is scarce. As a result, strategies for effective pain control in this population are based mostly on clinical experience and application of pain control methods shown to be useful with younger adults. There is a serious need for research in all areas of pain control for elders to identify adaptations in interventions useful to this population.

Pharmacologic Management

Although pharmacologic intervention might not be the sole intervention of choice for the older adult with chronic pain, it does have an important place in managing both malignant and benign chronic pain. In fact, analgesic use among elders has been shown to be prevalent (Chrischilles, Lemke, Wallace, & Drube, 1990; Thomas & Roy, 1988). However, a number of concerns are often noted related to the use of analgesic agents for elders that impact pharmacologic management. Concerns related to physiologic changes occurring with age, fears of addiction, seriousness of respiratory depression and other side effects, appropriateness of opioids for chronic pain, and problems related to compliance will be addressed.

Due to age-related physiologic changes affecting pharmacokinetics and pharmacodynamics, and problems of polypharmacy and idiosyncratic drug reactions, pharmacologic management of pain entails special considerations in elders (Butler & Gastel, 1980; B. A. Ferrell & B. R. Ferrell, 1991; Harkins et al., 1984; Portenoy & Farkash, 1988). In general, increases in the proportion of body fat, decreased circulating proteins, decreased hepatic metabolism, reduced glomerular filtration, and decreased drug clearance from plasma contribute to changes in response to pharmacologic intervention in the aged individual. The result of these physiological changes is increased sensitivity to the effect of analgesics, with a higher peak and longer duration of pain relief, as well as greater risk of toxic effect (Bellville, Forrest, Miller, & Brown, 1971; Kaiko, Wallenstein, Rogers, Grabinski, & Houde, 1982; Kwentus, Harkins, Lignon, & Silvermann, 1985; Moore, Vilderman, Lubenskyi, McCans, & Fox, 1990; Zaccharias, Pfeifer, & Herbison, 1990).

Although elders may be more sensitive to opioids, this does not justify withholding them and failing to treat their pain. Pharmacologic strategies are often less than adequate in controlling pain in elders primarily due to ineffective dosing and ineffective patterns of administration by both physicians and nurses (B. R. Ferrell et al., 1990; Roy & Thomas, 1986). The difference between the therapeutic dose of a medication and the toxic dose is smaller in elders requiring more careful monitoring. The potentially dangerous side effects of opioids, such as respiratory depression, can be monitored with careful and frequent assessments of the individual's response to the narcotic, and usually avoided by adjustment of the dose or interval between doses.

Concern over the use of opioids for the treatment of chronic pain in elders is generated primarily by an unreasonable fear of opiate addiction, a common concern of health care providers, older adults, and their families, that contributes to undertreatment of pain with opioids in this population (Faherty & Grier, 1984; McCaffery & Ferrell, 1991; Short, Burnett,

Egbert, & Parks, 1990). Contributing to the misconceptions of health professionals about the safe use of opioids is inadequate knowledge of pharmacology (McCaffery & Ferrell, 1991; McCaffery et al., 1990; Ryan, Vortherms, & Ward, 1994; Sheidler, McGuire, Gilbert, & Grossman, 1989). Studies conducted by B. R. Ferrell, McCaffrey, et al. (1992); B. R. Ferrell and B. A. Ferrell, (1993); and B. R. Ferrell, McGuire, et al. (1993) indicate that considerable inaccuracy exists in nursing texts concerning addiction, that faculty are confused about key principles of pharmacologic pain management, and educational efforts in this area are less than effective. Even less is evident in the gerontological literature.

Similarly, older adults themselves often have strong beliefs about the use of drugs. Many elders were raised in an era when "taking drugs" was the least preferred method of treatment. They have concerns about "becoming hooked on drugs" and "becoming an addict," often creating unreasonable fear that results in their unwillingness to try analgesics for the length of time that may be required to achieve therapeutic blood levels and to maintain pain relief.

Obviously unreasonable fears can seriously impact the adequacy of pain management and must be overcome. Research, however, indicates that addiction is rare with an incidence of less than 0.1% (Angel, 1982). Continued efforts must be made in professional education programs to correct misconceptions regarding the use of opioids with elders, as well as sharing accurate information with the patient and family to alleviate these fears.

A closely related concern is the belief that the potential for respiratory depression makes opioids too dangerous for use with elders. Although elders will require smaller doses of opioid to reduce the risk of opiate-induced respiratory depression (Caradoc-Davies, 1981), this serious side effect can be prevented by monitoring sedation and respiratory levels and appropriate dose titration in response to assessment findings.

Other side effects, including cognitive impairment, urinary retention, constipation, and intestinal obstruction, occur more frequently in elders population and need to be considered as well when intervening with opioids. Prevention is a key strategy to avoid and control these side effects and can be facilitated by careful dose titration and monitoring for early signs of occurrence. These side effects can be minimized by observing for signs of cognitive changes, assessing for irregularities in voiding, and initiating a bowel protocol. Although drug side effects can create significant problems for elders, concerns can be reduced if these are anticipated and treated vigorously.

Although a review of individual drugs and specific points of administration of opioid and nonopioid analgesics is beyond the scope of this chapter, several important generalizations will be addressed. Nonopioid analgesics, including acetaminophen and nonsteroidal anti-inflammatory drugs (NSAIDS), can be very effective and appropriate for use with elders either as adjuncts to opioids or as the sole pharmacologic intervention. NSAIDS are widely used by elders, especially for the treatment of arthritic conditions, which plague more than 80% of those 65 and older (Davis, 1988). However, the use of NSAIDS with elders requires special considerations. The risk for gastric and renal toxicity from NSAIDS is increased among elderly patients, and unusual drug reactions including cognitive impairment, constipation, and headaches also are more common (Roth, 1989). Because of these factors, the use of NSAIDS with the frail elderly requires caution and judicious monitoring. Careful evaluation of GI complaints is essential, and evaluation of hemoglobin/hematocrit and stool guaiac sample to monitor for GI bleed, and BUN and/or serum creatinine to screen for renal insufficiency should be conducted every 3 months.

Adjuvant medications, used to enhance analgesic effects, are often prescribed to treat chronic pain conditions. Antidepressants, anticonvulsants, sedative/antianxiety agents, steroids, muscle relaxants, and amphetamines often are used as adjuvant analgesics. These may be particularly useful for patients not responding to the usual pain protocol; however, there has been little in the way of research or guidelines relative to their use with elders and their effectiveness is sometimes unpredictable. Side effects with these agents are a big concern as well, since many are not treatable and are more frequent among elders (Salzman, 1984). Due to misperceptions related to the typical purpose of the drugs, careful explanations and education are important in promoting a positive response to these agents.

Because of the changes with aging mentioned earlier, there are some guidelines to follow when planning pharmacologic intervention with elders. Unless contraindicated by absorption problems or swallowing ability, oral medication should be used whenever possible. Drug absorption is highly variable and likely to be diminished in elders due to degenerated muscle from inactivity, poor nutrition, dehydration, and decreased peripheral circulation leading to insufficient plasma concentrations and delayed onset of action. If possible, intramuscular administration should be avoided, and other routes of administration, such as sublingual, buccal, rectal, subcutaneous, or intravenous, may be preferred.

The use of "high-tech" pain treatment, such as PCA or intraspinal analgesia, must be closely monitored and titrated carefully because of elders' increased sensitivity to drug effects (B. R. Ferrell, Cronin Nash, & Warfield, 1992). Although the use of patient-controlled analgesia (PCA) has been shown effective in elders with post-op pain (Duggleby & Lander, 1992; Egbert, Battit, Welch, & Barlett, 1990), no studies with cancer or other chronic pain conditions are available to document its effectiveness or the elders' ability to use the equipment correctly. The costs and benefits of technologic approaches must be weighed carefully, especially in light of Medicare and Medicaid payment restrictions (Whedon & Ferrell, 1991).

Finally, compliance with the pharmacologic regimen can be particularly problematic with elderly patients. A study by Austin and colleagues (1986) revealed that more than 50% of the elderly studied were not taking their prescribed pain medications appropriately. The complexity of the medication regimen may be a factor in the elders' ability to follow the intervention plan. Other factors found to result in undermedication or overdosing is lack of understanding regarding pain and its treatment by the patient or caregiver (B. R. Ferrell, Taylor, Grant, Fowler, & Corbisiero, 1993). The recent market influx of agents (NSAIDS) with single or twice daily dosing increases compliance but restricts flexibility in adjusting drug levels, a significant concern for those whose renal function and metabolism may be compromised (Nuki, 1990). The misbeliefs regarding pain management strategies that interfere with compliance with the prescribed intervention plan held by elders and their caregivers must be carefully addressed.

Nonpharmacologic Intervention

Use of nonpharmacologic interventions, in combination with pharmacologic approaches, can yield more positive outcomes for the client, including more effective pain control, less reliance on medications, fewer side effects, and less clinical impairment (B. A. Ferrell, 1991; Foley, 1990; McCaffery & Beebe, 1989; Middaugh, Levin, Kee, Barchiesi, & Roberts, 1988; Owens & Ehrenreich, 1991). Nonpharmacologic interventions can be classified in two ways. Physical or cutaneous stimulation interventions involve stimulating the skin and underlying tissues to moderate or relieve pain and include application of heat and cold, massage, and Transcutaneous Electrical Nerve Stimulation (TENS) among others. Cognitive-behavioral interventions focus on helping the individual cope with the pain being experienced by altering the interpretation of the sensation of pain and enhancing self-control. These strategies include cognitive therapy, relaxation, imagery, distraction, hypnosis, and biofeedback.

Although many pain specialists, and a growing number of geriatricians, advocate the use of nonpharmacologic interventions for elderly clients (Butler & Gastel, 1980; B. A. Ferrell, 1991; Harkins et al., 1984; Hunt, 1980; Kwentus et al., 1985), many health care providers perceive older adults as indifferent, unwilling, or unable to use nonpharmacologic interventions; however, empirical evidence reveals that older patients are often very responsive to the use of these interventions. In a study comparing characteristics of younger and older chronic pain patients, Sorkin et al. (1990) found that older adults were equally as likely to report the use of physical nonpharmacologic techniques for pain relief (e.g., TENS, heat, and massage), but were less likely to report use of cognitive-behavioral techniques (e.g., relaxation, imagery, distraction) than their younger counterparts. Of importance, however, was the finding that elder clients were as likely as younger clients to accept and complete treatments involving both physical and cognitive-behavioral strategies when offered. This supports the contention that age should not be a significant consideration when offering clients multimodal treatment strategies for pain, including both cognitive-behavioral as well as physical nonpharmacologic modalities.

Similarly, in a study of the responses of geriatric and younger clients to a multidisciplinary chronic pain rehabilitation program offering both physical and cognitive-behavioral interventions, Middaugh et al. (1988) found that geriatric clients can benefit from these programs at least as much as, if not more than, younger clients. Further, they note that geriatric clients often show greater interest in these programs, are more compliant than their younger counterparts, are more willing to work hard for degrees of improvement, and are generally free of the work-related issues that hinder progress for younger patients.

Because pharmacologic interventions often are the primary strategy for managing pain, the majority of health professionals may not be aware of the value of incorporating nonpharmacologic strategies into the treatment regimen and may lack sufficient knowledge to use them effectively. In a study of medical, surgical, and oncology nurses, Dalton (1989) found that nonpharmacologic interventions were familiar to the nurses studied, although they reported using most of them less than 25% of the time. Edgar and Smith-Hanrahan (1992) propose that this may be due, at least in part, to a lack of adequate knowledge or skills necessary for implementation of these interventions. Incorporation of the content related to the use of these techniques into health professional curricula should increase the use of nonpharmacologic strategies with the older adult in pain.

As with all treatment modalities, there are individual differences in the acceptance and use of nonpharmacologic interventions that must be considered. Cognitive-behavioral strategies, in particular, require clients to have a greater degree of self-efficacy with respect to managing their pain and often require continuous effort by the client to be effective. Additionally, cognitive-behavioral interventions such as relaxation and imagery require high levels of cognitive function to be used effectively. Other factors that are important in the selection of interventions for managing pain include the pathophysiologic basis of the pain, functional status, social and financial support, and developed coping strategies (B. A. Ferrell & B. R. Ferrell, 1991; Portenoy & Farkash, 1988).

Available research, though limited, supports the use and effectiveness of both cutaneous stimulation and cognitive-behavioral nonpharmacologic interventions for elders. Although discussion of the research to date is beyond the scope of this chapter, interested readers are referred to a number of publications describing, in greater detail, the clinical use and empirical review of nonpharmacologic interventions with elders (Edgar & Smith-Hanrahan, 1992; B. A. Ferrell, 1991; B. A. Ferrell & B. R. Ferrell, 1991; McCaffery & Beebe, 1989; Mobily, 1994; Saxon, 1991).

The empirical bases for the use of nonpharmacologic interventions have been well researched in younger populations; however, additional research with older adults is needed to evaluate process and outcome measures, to determine the most effective clinical approaches for this population, and to evaluate cost-effectiveness and long-term outcomes.

Despite the obvious benefits of using nonpharmacologic interventions, these are adjunctive therapies, and, for most acute and chronic pain problems, these are not substitutes for pharmacologic treatment. Optimal management of chronic pain in older adults is achieved through use of both pharmacologic and nonpharmacologic strategies.

Financial Considerations

Selecting appropriate interventions for managing pain in elders can be a daunting challenge in this age of cost containment. Technological advances that provide increased options for control of severe pain, including sustained release oral and transdermal preparations, patient-controlled analgesic devices, and intraspinal opioid infusion systems, are available. Cost, however, can be an overriding factor when evaluating the benefits of these options for use with elders. Because the research to support the effectiveness of many of these advances with elders population does not exist, their use is questioned, especially by third-party payers. Because of the increased scrutiny of health care costs by governmental and private insurers, limitations and restrictions on health care costs impact the strategies that can be selected. Denying coverage of certain techniques (epidural catheters), denying reimbursement for the use of equipment (such as TENS and patient-controlled analgesia pumps), questioning the prescription of certain medications (in particular, long-term use of opioids), and limited reimbursement for services provided in the home setting can all affect the effectiveness of pain management with elders.

Nurses need to involve themselves in reimbursement and financial issues. The profession can play a key role in determining the future direction of pain management for elders. It is our role to serve as an advocate to determine the best treatment plan, to consider the impact of technology on the patient's quality of life, to examine the monetary as well as quality of life issues related to use of technological equipment, and to conduct the research needed to determine its clinical and cost-effectiveness with elders.

INTEGRATED APPROACH TO PAIN MANAGEMENT

Management of pain in elders population has become a very complex task. The older adult with chronic pain is best served through the efforts of an interdisciplinary team that collaborates through regular communications and planning sessions to achieve desired outcomes. Because professional nursing education does include skills in communication, collaboration, negotiation, and leadership, the nurse often is in the best position to serve as the manager of care for these individuals.

Another opportunity for collaborative care is in the referral of older adults with chronic pain to multidisciplinary rehabilitation programs for evaluation and treatment recommendations. Although the incidence of chronic pain is obviously high, few elderly individuals attend multidisciplinary clinics for treatment of chronic pain (Harkins, 1988; Roy, 1987). Evaluation of rehabilitation programs to treat chronic pain has demonstrated that geriatric patients can benefit from these programs at least as much as, if not more than, younger patients (Middaugh et al., 1988; Sorkin et al.,

1990). Pain center referral is probably appropriate for the majority of older chronic pain patients with significant functional and psychological impairments (Portenoy & Farkash, 1988) and should be considered for selected elders. Once again, financial considerations with respect to cost and reimbursement are important, but must be weighed against costly negative outcomes of no treatment, such as loss of functional independence, increased caregiver burden, increased need for institutionalization, and decreased quality of life.

SUMMARY

Most of the older population suffer from at least one chronic condition that can cause considerable pain and impact quality of life. Although research to document this relationship is limited, clinical observation suggests the problems created by pain in elders are considerable. Pain, discomfort, and suffering must no longer be accepted as a normal consequence of growing old.

The evaluation of treatments in controlled studies as well as the implementation and evaluation of interventions in clinical care require an accurate assessment of clinical pain. Given the potential impact of pain in this population, it is critical that health care providers carefully and systematically evaluate any pain complaint. The special needs of those unable to communicate for themselves must also be considered as we address the treatment of elders. Older adults experiencing chronic pain need the advocacy of family, health care professionals, and professional organizations to make their pain visible and to assure that comfort is given a high priority.

A multimodal approach incorporating both pharmacologic and nonpharmacologic strategies is indicated for effective management of pain in elders. Educational efforts should be directed toward the health care professional, as well as the patient and family, regarding the special concerns with pain management for the older adult.

Despite the continuing growth of this segment of our population, research examining the effects of age on various pain control modalities is scarce. As a result, strategies for effective pain control in this population are at present based mostly on clinical experience and application of pain control methods shown to be useful with younger adults. There is a serious need for research in all areas of pain control for elders to identify adaptations in intervention useful for this population. Through research, a more comprehensive, rational, scientifically based process of pain management will be possible and the quality of life of older adults will be enhanced.

REFERENCES

Acute Pain Management Guideline Panel. (1992). *Acute pain management: Operative or medical procedures and trauma. Clinical practice guideline* (AHCPR Pub. No. 92-0032). Rockville, MD: Agency for Health Care Policy and Research, U.S. Department of Health and Human Services, Public Health Service.

Angel, M. (1982). The quality of mercy. *New England Journal of Medicine, 306,* 98–99.

Beck, A. T., Ward, C., Mendelson, M., Mock, J., & Erbaugh, J. (1961). An inventory for measuring depression. *Archives of General Psychiatry, 4,* 561–571.

Bellville, J. W., Forrest, W. H., Miller, E., & Brown, B. W. (1971). Influence of age on pain relief from analgesics. *Journal of the American Medical Association, 217*(13), 1835–1841.

Bender, J. (1989). Approach to the acute abdomen. *Medical Clinics of North America, 73,* 1413–1422.

Beyer, J. E., & Aradine, C. R. (1986). Content validity of an instrument to measure young children's perceptions of the intensity of their pain. *Journal of Pediatric Nursing, 1,* 386–395.

Bieri, D., Reeve, R., Champion, G., Addicoat, L., & Ziegler, J. (1990). The Faces Pain Scale for the self-assessment of the severity of pain experienced by children: Development, initial validation, and preliminary investigation for ratio scale properties. *Pain, 41,* 139–150.

Blazer, D., Hughes, D., & George, L. (1987). The epidemiology of depression in an elderly community population. *Gerontologist, 27,* 281–287.

Blumer, D., & Heilbronn, M. (1981). The pain-prone disorder: A clinical and psychological profile. *Psychosomatics, 22,* 395–402.

Bonica, J. J. (1990). General considerations of chronic pain. In J. J. Bonica (Ed.), *The management of pain* (2nd ed., pp. 180–196). Philadephia: Lea and Febiger.

Brattberg, G., Mats, T., & Anders, W. (1989). The prevalence of pain in a general population: The results of a postal survey in a county of Sweden. *Pain, 37,* 215–222.

Brody, E. M., & Kleban, M. H. (1983). Day-to-day mental and physical health symptoms of older people: A report on health logs. *Gerontologist, 23,* 75–85.

Brown, G., Nicassio, P., & Wallston, K. (1989). Pain coping strategies and depression in rheumatoid arthritis. *Journal of Consulting and Clinical Psychology, 57,* 652–657.

Brunier, G., Carson, G., & Harrison, D. (1995). What do nurses know and believe about patients with pain? Results of a hospital survey. *Journal of Pain and Symptom Management, 10*(6), 436–445.

Butler, R. H., & Gastel, B. (1980). Care of the aged: Perspectives of pain and discomfort. In L. K. Ng & J. J. Bonica (Eds.), *Pain, discomfort and humanitarian care.* Proceedings of the National Conference, Bethesda, MD, February 15–16, 1979. New York: Elsevier.

Caradoc-Davies, T. H. (1981). Opiate toxicity in elderly patients. *British Medical Journal, 283,* 823–826.

Chapman, C. R., & Syrjala, K .L. (1990). Measurement of pain. In J. J. Bonica (Ed.), *The management of pain* (2nd ed., pp. 580–594). Philadelphia: Lea and Febriger.

Chrischilles, E., Lemke, J., Wallace, R., & Drube, G. (1990). Prevalence and characteristics of multiple analgesic drug use in an elderly study group. *Journal of the American Geriatrics Society, 38,* 979–984.

Closs, S. José. (1994). Pain in elderly patients: A neglected phenomenon? *Journal of Advanced Nursing, 19,* 1072–1081.

Copp, L. A. (1990). The spectrum of suffering. *American Journal of Nursing, 90*(8), 35–39.

Craig, K. D., Hyde, S. A., & Patrick, C. J. (1991). Genuine, suppressed and faked facial behavioural exacerbation of chronic low back pain. *Pain, 46,* 153–160.

Crook, J., Rideout, E., & Browne, G. (1984). The prevalence of pain complaints among a general population. *Pain, 18,* 299–314.

Dalton, J. (1989). Nurses' perceptions of their pain assessment skills, pain management practices, and attitudes toward pain. *Oncology Nursing Forum, 16*(2), 225–231.

Dastoor, D., Schwartz, G., & Kurzman, D. (1991). Clock-drawing—An assessment technique in dementia. *Journal of Clinical and Experimental Gerontology, 13*(1–2), 69–85.

Davis, M. E. (1988). Epidemiology of osteoarthritism. *Clinics in Geriatric Medicine, 4,* 241–255.

Demlow, L., Liang, M., & Eaton, H. (1986). Impact of chronic arthritis on the elderly. *Clinics in Rheumatic Diseases, 12,* 329–335.

Diekmann, J., & Wassem, R. (1991). A survey of nursing students' knowledge of cancer pain control. *Cancer Nursing, 14,* 314–320.

Doan, B., & Wadden, N. (1989). Relationships between depressive symptoms and description of chronic pain. *Pain, 36,* 75–84.

Donovan, M. (1989). Relieving pain: The current bases for practice. In S. Funk,

E. Tornquist, M. Champagne, L. Copp, & R. Wiese (Eds.), *Key aspects of comfort: Management of pain, fatigue, and nausea* (pp. 25–34). New York: Springer.

Duggleby, W., & Lander, J. (1992). Patient-controlled analgesia for older adults. *Clinical Nursing Research, 1*(1), 107–113.

Edgar, L., & Smith-Hanrahan, C. (1992). Nonpharmacologic pain management. In J. H. Watt-Watson & M. I. Donovan (Eds.), *Pain management: Nursing perspective* (pp. 162–202). St. Louis: Mosby.

Egbert, L. D., Battit, G. E., Welch, C. E., & Barlett, M. K. (1990). Randomized trial of postoperative patient controlled analgesia vs intramuscular narcotics in frail elderly men. *Archives of Internal Medicine, 150,* 1897–1903.

Enck, R. (1991). Pain control in the ambulatory elderly. *Geriatrics, 46*(3), 49–53, 57–58a, 60.

Faherty, B. S., & Grier, M. R. (1984). Analgesic medication for elderly people post-surgery. *Nursing Research, 33*(6), 369–372.

Ferrell, B. A. (1991). Pain management in elderly people. *Journal of the American Geriatrics Society, 39,* 64–73.

Ferrell, B. A., & Ferrell, B. R. (1991). Principles of pain management in older people. *Comprehensive Therapy, 17,* 53.

Ferrell, B. A., Ferrell, B. R., & Osterweil, D. (1990). Pain in the nursing home. *Journal of the American Geriatrics Society, 38*(4), 409–414.

Ferrell, B. R., Cronin Nash, C., & Warfield, C. (1992). The role of patient-controlled analgesia in the management of cancer pain. *Journal of Pain and Symptom Management, 7*(3), 149–154.

Ferrell, B. R., & Ferrell, B. A. (1992). Pain in the elderly. In J. Watt-Watson & M. I. Donovan (Eds.), *Pain* (pp. 349–369). St. Louis: Mosby.

Ferrell, B. R., Grant, M., Padilla, G.,Vemuri, S., & Rhiner, M. (1991). The experience of pain and perceptions of quality of life: Validation of a conceptual model. *Hospice Journal, 7,* 79–124.

Ferrell, B. R., McCaffery, M., & Rhiner, M. (1992). Pain and addiction: An urgent need for change in nursing education. *Journal of Pain and Symptom Management, 7*(2), 117–124.

Ferrell, B. R., McGuire, D., & Donovan, M. (1993). Knowledge and beliefs of nursing faculty regarding pain. *Journal of Professional Nursing, 9*(2), 79–88.

Ferrell, B. R., Taylor, E. J., Grant, M., Fowler, M., & Corbisiero, R. (1993). Pain management at home. Struggle, comfort and mission. *Cancer Nursing, 16,* 169–178.

Ferrell, B. R., Wisdom, C., & Wenzel, C. (1989). Quality of life as an outcome variable in the management of cancer pain. *Cancer, 63,* 2321–2327.

Ferrell, B. R., Wisdom, C., Wenzel, C., & Brown, J. (1990). Controlled release vs. short acting analgesia: Effects on pain and quality of life. *Oncology Nursing Forum, 26,* 521–526.

Foley, K. (1985). Treatment of cancer pain. *New England Journal of Medicine, 113,* 84–95.

Foley, K. M. (1990). Pain management in elders. In R. Andres, E. L. Bierman, & J. P. Blass (Eds.), *Principles of geriatric medicine.* New York: McGraw-Hill.

Folstein, M. F., Folstein, S. A., & McHugh, P. R. (1975). Mini Mental State: A practical method for grading the cognitive state of patients for the clinician. *Journal of Psychiatric Research, 12,* 189–198.

Gordon, R. S. (1979). Pain in the elderly. *Journal of the American Medical Association, 24,* 2191.

Graffam, S. (1990). Pain content in the curriculum—A survey. *Nurse Educator, 15*(1), 20–23.

Guccione, A. A., Meenan, R. F., & Anderson, J. J. (1989). Arthritis in nursing home residents: A validation of its prevalence and examination of its impact on institutionalization and functional status. *Arthritis and Rheumatism, 32*(12), 1546–1553.

Haley, W., Turner, J., & Romano, J. (1985). Depression and chronic pain patients: Relation to pain, activity, and sex differences. *Pain, 23,* 337–343.

Haley, W. E., & Dolce, J. J. (1986). Assessment and management of chronic pain in elders. *Clinical Gerontologist, 5*(3/4), 435–455.

Harkins, S. (1988). Pain in the elderly. In R. Dubner, G. F. Gebhart, & M. R. Bond (Eds.), *Proceedings of the 5th World Congress on Pain* (pp. 355–367). New York: Elsevier.

Harkins, S., Price, D., & Martelli, M. (1986). Effects of age on pain perception: Thermonociception. *Journal of Gerontology, 41*(1), 58–63.

Harkins, S. W., & Chapman, C. R. (1976). Detection and decision factors in pain perception in young and elderly men. *Pain, 2,* 253.

Harkins, S. W., & Chapman, C. R. (1977). The perception of induced dental pain in young and elderly women. *Journal of Gerontology, 32,* 428–435.

Harkins, S. W., Kwentus, J., & Price, D. D. (1984). Pain and the elderly. In C. Benedetti, C. R. Chapman, & G. Moricca (Eds.), *Advances in pain research and therapy: Vol. 7* (pp. 103–122). New York: Raven Press.

Haythornthwaite, J., Seiber, W., & Kerns, R. (1991). Depression and the chronic pain experience. *Pain, 46,* 177–184.

Herr, K., & Mobily, P. (1991). Complexities of pain assessment in elders: Clinical considerations. *Journal of Gerontological Nursing, 17*(4), 12–19.

Herr, K., & Mobily, P. (1992). Geriatric mental health: Chronic pain and depression. *Journal of Psychosocial Nursing, 30*(9), 7–12.

Herr, K., Mobily, P., & Smith, C. (1993). Depression and the experience of chronic back pain: A study of related variables and age differences. *Clinical Journal of Pain, 9,* 104–114.

Herr, K., Mobily, P., Wallace, R., & Chung, Y. (1991). Leg pain in the rural Iowa

65+ population: Prevalence, related factors and association with functional status. *Clinical Journal of Pain, 7,* 114–121.

Hickey, T. (1988). Changing health perceptions of older patients and the implications for assessment. *Geriatric Medicine Today, 7*(6), 59–66.

Hofland, S. L. (1992). Elder beliefs: Blocks to pain management. *Journal of Gerontological Nursing, 18*(6), 19–24, 39–40.

Hunt, T. E. (1980). Pain and the aged patient. In W. L. Smith, H. Merskey, & S. C. Gross (Eds.), *Pain, meaning and management* (pp. 143–158). Jamaica, NY: Spectrum.

Hurley, A. C., Volicer, B. J., Hanrahan, P. A., Houde, S., & Volicer, L. (1992). Assessment of discomfort in advanced Alzheimer patients. *Research in Nursing and Health, 15,* 369–377.

Jacobs, J., Bernhard, M., Delgado, A., & Strain, J. (1977). Screening for organic mental syndromes in the medically ill. *Annals of Internal Medicine, 86,* 40–46.

Jacox, A., Carr, D. B., Payne, R., et al. (1994). *Management of cancer pain. Clinical practice guideline No. 9* (AHCPR Pub. No. 94–0592). Rockville, MD: Agency for Health Care Policy and Research, U.S. Department of Health and Human Services, Public Health Service.

Jay, L., & Miller, T. (1990). Chronic pain and the geriatric patient. In T. Miller (Ed.), *Chronic pain: Vol. 2* (pp. 821–838). Madison, WI: International Universities Press.

Jensen, M. P., Karoly, P., & Braver, S. (1986). The measurement of clinical pain intensity: A comparison of six methods. *Pain, 27,* 117–126.

Kaiko, R. F., Wallenstein, S. L., Rogers, A. G., Grabinski, P. Y., & Houde, R. W. (1982). Narcotics in the elderly. *Medical Clinics of North America, 66*(5), 1079–1089.

Katz, S., Ford, A. B., Moskowitz, R. W., Jackson, B. A., & Jaffe, M. W. (1963). Studies of illness in the aged. The index of activities of daily living: A standardized measure of biological and psychological function. *Journal of the American Medical Association, 185,* 914–919.

Keefe, F., Wilkins, R., Cook, W., Crisson, J., & Muhlbaier, L. (1986). Depression, pain and pain behavior. *Journal of Consulting and Clinical Psychology, 54,* 665–669.

Kerns, R., & Turk, D. (1984). Depression and chronic pain: The mediating role of the spouse. *Journal of Marriage and Family, 46,* 845–852.

Kerns, R., Turk, D., & Rudy, T. (1985). The West Haven-Yale Multidimensional Pain Inventory (WHYMPI). *Pain, 23,* 345–356.

Kleinke, C., & Spangler, A. (1988). Predicting treatment outcome of chronic back pain patients in a multidisciplinary pain clinic: Methodological issues and treatment implications. *Pain, 33,* 41–48.

Kotler-Cope, S., & Gerber, K. E. (1993). Is age related to response to treatment for chronic pain? *Abstracts of the 7th World Congress on Pain.* Seattle, WA: International Association for the Study of Pain.

Kremer, E., Atkinson, J. H., & Ignelzi, R. J. (1981). Measurement of pain: Patient preference does not confound pain measurement. *Pain, 10,* 241–249.

Kwentus, J. A., Harkins, S. W., Lignon, N., & Silvermann, J. J. (1985). Current concepts of geriatric pain and its treatment. *Geriatrics, 40*(4), 48–57.

Lau-Ting, C., & Phoon, W. O. (1988). Ache and pains among Singapore elderly. *Singapore Medical Journal, 29,* 164–167.

Lavsky-Shulan, M., Wallace, R. B., Kohout, F. J., Lemke, J. H., Morris, M. C., & Smith, I. M. (1985). Prevalence and functional correlates of low back pain in the elderly: The Iowa 65+ rural health study. *Journal of the American Geriatrics Society, 33*(1), 23–28.

Lawton, M. P., & Brody, E. M. (1969). Assessment of older people: Self-maintaining and instrumental activities of daily living. *Gerontologist, 9,* 179–186.

Liang , M. H., Larson, M., Thompson, M., Eaton, H., McNamara, E., Katz, R., & Taylor, J. (1984). Costs and outcomes in rheumatoid arthritis and osteoarthritis. *Arthritis and Rheumatism, 27,* 864–872.

Liebeskind, J. C., & Melzack, R. (1987). The International Pain Foundation: Meeting a need for education in pain management. *Pain, 30,* 1–2.

Magni, G., Schifano, F., & DeLeo, D. (1985). Pain as a symptom in elderly depressed patients: Relationship to diagnostic subgroups. *European Archives of Psychiatry and Clinical Neuroscience, 235,* 143–145.

Mahoney, F., & Barthel, D. (1965). Functional evaluation: The Barthel Index. *MS Medical Journal, 14*(2), 61–65.

Marks, R. M., & Sachar, E. J. (1973). Undertreatment of medical inpatients with narcotic analgesia. *Annals of Internal Medicine, 78,* 173–181.

Marzinski, L. (1991). The tragedy of dementia: Clinically assessing pain in the confused, nonverbal elderly. *Journal of Gerontological Nursing, 17*(6), 25–28.

McCaffery, M., & Beebe, A. (1989). *Pain: Clinical manual for nursing practice.* St. Louis: Mosby.

McCaffery, M., & Ferrell, B. (1991). How would you respond to these patients in pain? *Nursing, 91*(6), 34–37.

McCaffery, M., & Ferrell, B. (1992). Opioid analgesics: Nurses' knowledge of doses and psychological dependence. *Journal of Nursing Staff Development, 8* (March/April), 77–84.

McCaffery, M., Ferrell, B. R., O'Neil-Page, E., Lester, M., & Ferrell, B. A. (1990). Nurses' knowledge of opioid analgesic drugs and psychological dependence. *Cancer Nursing, 13*(20), 21–27.

McGrath, P. A., DeVeber, L. L., & Hearn, M. T. (1985). Multidimensional pain assessment in children. In H. L. Field, R. Dubner, & F. Cevero (Eds.), *Advances in pain research and therapy* (pp. 387–393). New York: Raven Press.

Melding, P. (1991). Is there such a thing as geriatric pain? *Pain, 46,* 119–121.

Melzack, R., & Wall, P. D. (1965). Pain mechanisms: A new theory. *Science, 150,* 971–979.

Melzack, R., & Wall, P. D. (1982). *The puzzle of pain.* New York: Basic Books.

Middaugh, S., Levin, R., Kee, W., Barchiesi, F., & Roberts, J. (1988). Chronic pain: Its treatment in geriatric and younger patients. *Archives of Physical Medicine and Rehabilitation, 69,* 1021–1026.

Mobily, P. (1994). Nonpharmacologic interventions for the management of chronic pain in older women. *Journal of Women and Aging, 6*(4), 89–109.

Mobily, P., Herr, K., Clark, M. K., & Wallace, R. (1994). An epidemiologic analysis of pain in the elderly. *Journal of Aging and Health, 6*(2), 139–154.

Moore, A. K., Vilderman, S., Lubenskyi, W., McCans, J., & Fox, G. S. (1990). Differences in epidural morphine requirements between elderly and young patients after abdominal surgery. *Anesthesia and Analgesia, 70,* 316–320.

Moss, M. A., Lawton, M. P., & Glicksman, A. (1991). The role of pain in the last year of life of older persons. *Journal of Gerontology: Psychological Sciences, 46*(2), 51–57.

Nuki, G. (1990). Pain control and the use of non-steroidal antiinflammatory drugs. *British Medical Journal, 46*(1), 262–278.

Owens, M. K., & Ehrenreich, D. (1991). Literature review of nonpharmacologic methods for the treatment of chronic pain. *Holistic Nursing Practice, 6*(1), 24–31.

Parmalee, P., Katz, I., & Lawton, M. (1991). The relation of pain to depression among institutionalized aged. *Journal of Gerontology: Psychological Sciences, 46,* 15–21.

Parmalee, P. A., Smith, B., & Katz, I. R. (1993). Pain complaints and cognitive status among elderly institution residents. *Journal of the American Geriatrics Society, 41,* 517–522.

Pfeiffer, E. (1975). A short portable mental status questionnaire for the assessment of organic brain deficit in elderly patients. *Journal of the American Geriatric Society, 23,* 433–441.

Portenoy, R. K. (1988). Drug treatment of pain syndromes. *Seminars of Neurology, 7*(2), 139–149.

Portenoy, R. K. (1993, January). Drug therapy for neuropathic pain. *Drug Therapy, 7,* 41.

Portenoy, R. K., & Farkash, A. (1988). Practical management of non-malignant pain in the elderly. *Geriatrics, 43*(5), 29–47.

Prkachin, K. M. (1992). The consistency of facial expressions of pain: A comparison across modalities. *Pain, 51,* 297–306.

Radloff, L. (1977). The CES-D Scale: A self-report depression scale for research in the general population. *Applied Psychological Measurement, 1*(3), 385–401.

Rankin, M., & Snider, B. (1984). Nurses' perceptions of cancer patients' pain. *Cancer Nursing, 11,* 203–209.

Romano, J., & Turner, J. (1985). Chronic pain and depression: Does the evidence support a relationship? *Psychological Bulletin, 97,* 18–34.

Rosenstiel, A. K., & Keefe, F. J. (1983). The use of coping strategies in chronic low back pain patients: Relationship to patient characteristics and current adjustments. *Pain, 17,* 33–44.

Roth, S. H. (1989). Merits and liabilities of NSAID therapy. *Rheumatic Diseases Clinics of North America, 15,* 479–498.

Rousseau, P., & Calvin, P. (1993). Nurses' interpretation of pain in long-term care facilities. *Journal of Medical Direction, 3*(1), 28–29.

Roy, R. (1987). A psychosocial perspective on chronic pain and depression in the elderly. *Social Work in Health Care, 12,* 1227–1236.

Roy, R., & Thomas, M. R. (1986). A survey of chronic pain in an elderly population. *Canadian Family Physician, 32,* 513–516.

Roy, R., & Thomas, M. R. (1987). Elderly persons with and without pain: A comparative study. *Clinical Journal of Pain, 3,* 102–106.

Rudy, T., Kerns, R., & Turk, D. (1988). Chronic pain and depression: Toward a cognitive-behavioral mediation model. *Pain, 35,* 129–140.

Ryan, P., Vortherms, R., & Ward, S. (1994). Cancer pain: Knowledge, attitudes of pharmacologic management. *Journal of Gerontological Nursing, 20*(1), 7–16.

Salzman, C. (1984). *Clinical geriatric psycho-pharmacology.* New York: McGraw-Hill.

Saxon, S. (1991). *Pain management techniques for older adults.* Springfield, IL: Charles C. Thomas.

Shapiro, B., & Ferrell, B. R. (1992, October). Pain in children and the frail elderly: Similarities and implications. *APS Bulletin, 2,* 11–13.

Sheidler, V., McGuire, D., Gilbert, M., & Grossman, S. (1989). Nurses' (RNs) inabilities to recognize safe narcotics orders. *Oncology Nursing Forum, 16*(2), 195. (Suppl.)

Sheidler, V., McGuire, D., Grossman, S., & Gilbert, M. (1992). Analgesic decision-making skills of nurses. *Oncology Nursing Forum, 19,* 1531–1534.

Short, L. M., Burnett, M. S., Egbert, A. M., & Parks, L. H. (1990). Medicating the postoperative elderly: How do nurses make their decisions? *Journal of Gerontological Nursing, 16*(7), 12–17.

Shulman, K., Shedletsky, R., & Silver, I. (1986). The challenge of time: Clock-drawing and cognitive function in the elderly. *International Journal of Geriatric Psychiatry, 1,* 135–140.

Sorkin, B., Rudy, R., Hanlon, R., Turk, D., & Stieg, R. (1990). Chronic pain in old and young patients: Differences appear less important than similarities. *Journal of Gerontology: Psychological Sciences, 45,* 64–68.

Tait, R. C. (1993). Management of pain in the elderly. In P. A. Szwabo & G. T. Grossberg (Eds.), *Problem behaviors in long-term care: Recognition, diagnosis & treatment.* New York: Springer.

Tait, R., Pollard, C., Margolis, R., Duckro, P., & Krause, S. (1987). The Pain Disability Index: Psychometric and validity data. *Archives of Physical and Medical Rehabilitation, 68,* 438–441.

Teske, K., Daut, R., & Cleeland, C. (1983). Relationships between nurses' observations and patients' self-reports of pain. *Pain, 16,* 289–296.

Thomas, M. R., & Roy, R. (1988). Age and pain: A comparative study of the younger and older elderly. *Pain Management, 1,* 174–179.

Tucker, M. A., Andrew, M. F., Ogle, S. J., & Davison, J. G. (1989). Age associated change in pain threshold measured by transcutaneous neuronal electrical stimulation. *Age and Ageing, 18,* 241–246.

Turk, D., Okifuji, A., & Scharff, L. (1994). Assessment of older women with chronic pain. *Journal of Women & Aging, 6*(4), 25–42.

Turk, D. C., Kerns, R. D., & Rosenberg, R. (1992). Effects of marital interaction on chronic pain and disability: Examining the down-side of social support. *Rehabilitation Psychology, 37,* 259–274.

Tyler, D., Tu, A., Douthit, J., & Chapman, C. R. (1993). Toward validation of pain measurement tools for children: A pilot study. *Pain, 52,* 301–309.

Walker, J., Akinsanya, J., Davis, B., & Marcer, D. (1990). The nursing management of elderly patients with pain in the community: Study and recommendations. *Journal of Advanced Nursing, 15,* 1154–1161.

Wallace, K., Reed, B., Pasero, C., & Olsson, G. (1995). Staff nurses' perceptions of barriers to effective pain management. *Journal of Pain and Symptom Management, 10*(3), 204–213.

Watt-Watson, J., & Watson, C. (1989). Pain curriculum. *Canadian Nurse, 85*(9), 44–45.

Whedon, M., & Ferrell, B. R. (1991). Professional and ethical considerations in the use of high-tech pain management. *Oncology Nursing Forum, 18,* 1135–1143.

Williamson, G. M., & Schulz, R. (1992). Pain, activity restriction, and symptoms of depression among community-residing elderly adults. *Journal of Gerontology, 47*(6), 370–372.

Witte, M. (1989). Pain control. *Journal of Gerontological Nursing, 15*(3), 32–37.

Wolf-Klein, G., Silverstone, F., Levy, A., Brod, M., & Breuer, J. (1989). Screening for Alzheimer's disease by clock drawing. *Journal of the American Geriatric Society, 37,* 730–734.

Yesavage, J., Brink, T., Rose, T., Lum, O., Huang, V., Adey, M., & Leirer, V. (1983). Development and validation of a geriatric screening scale: A preliminary report. *Journal of Psychiatric Research, 17,* 37–49.

Zaccharias, M., Pfeifer, M. V., & Herbison, P. (1990). Comparison of two methods of intravenous administration of morphine for post-operative pain relief. *Anaesthesia and Intensive Care, 18,* 205–209.

CHAPTER **5**

Ethnicity, Aging, and Chronic Illness

Toni Tripp-Reimer

Elders who have lived as members of an ethnic group often acquire from that experience basic beliefs, practices, and expectations regarding aging, health, and illness. Yet, despite a considerable body of knowledge documenting the significance of ethnicity for both the experience of aging and chronic disorders, only in the past few years has serious attention been given to the interrelationships of these domains. In part, this inattention resulted from the American myth of the "melting pot." This myth emerged from a cultural ideal of equality coupled with a European ethnocentric perspective. The myth promoted the notion that all Americans are alike; however, the modal types for similarity were middle-class persons of European descent. For many years, the notion that ethnicity should be discounted was prominent in nursing and other health professions. However, the importance of ethnicity has recently been advocated by a small, but growing, component of multidisciplinary scientists in ethnogerontology. These ethnogerontologists typically are social or health scientists interested in the multiple reciprocal relationships among ethnic factors and the experience of aging.

Before discussing the relationships among ethnicity, aging, and chronic illness, it is important to clarify meanings. In discussions of ethnic elders, a variety of terms are employed in the literature, including culture, race, ethnic groups of color, minorities, and immigrants. The term "ethnicity" is preferred for this chapter because it is a broader term that encompasses variations based on any of the following: national origin (Greek), race (black), religion (Jewish), language (Hispanic).

Chronic illness, aging, and ethnicity are highly dynamic and interrelated concepts. The distinctive life patterns that characterize an ethnic group are salient for elders in several ways. This chapter will delineate some ways in which ethnicity can be expected to mediate the experiences of elders with chronic disorders. Included will be some of the ways in which ethnicity influences the distribution of disorders in a population, the ways in which symptoms are interpreted and illness is defined, patterns of lay and professional consultation, and access to and utilization of various treatment options. Ethnicity is also a critical variable in how the elder with the chronic disorder is perceived and treated by the family, and how the family, in turn, is viewed by the community at large. Cultural factors mediate the ways in which symptoms are identified and interpreted, the appropriate modes of the expression of pain and suffering, whether the illness is stigmatized or accepted, and whether the dependency that accompanies chronic illness is disvalued or considered a part of the normal life cycle (Tripp-Reimer & Lauer, 1987). Because elders are often the most traditionalist emboss of their ethnic group, these issues often have the greatest salience in their care.

Because of the diverse origins of people in the United States, there is greater heterogeneity among Americans than in most other Western cultures. While ethnicity is an important concept, it is critical to remember that none of the group characteristics (whether cultural or physical) that are used to denote ethnicity sharply distinguish any single population group. Additionally, it is important to recognize the significance of intraethnic diversity. Knowledge that there is as much variation within groups as between them will mitigate the tendency of health professionals and others to stereotype members of ethnic groups.

DEMOGRAPHIC PATTERNS

While many are aware that the proportion of elders is increasing faster than the general population in the United States, fewer recognize that minority elders are growing at even a more rapid rate than the general elder population. In the upcoming decades, there will be a dramatic increase in the proportion of ethnic elders. In 1990, the overwhelming majority of elders (87%) was white; however, this proportion is projected to decrease to 78% by 2020 and 67% by 2050. The proportion of black elders is projected to increase from 8% in 1990 to 10% in 2050. The proportion of Hispanic and

Asian elders is projected to increase much more rapidly. Hispanic elders are expected to increase from 4% in 1990 to 9% in 2020 and 16% in 2050. Similarly, Asian elders are likely to increase from 1% in 1990 to 8% in 2050. The largest proportionate increase is projected to occur in the over 75 age group, and this trend is more accelerated for minority elderly than for whites (U.S. Bureau of the Census, 1993).

Intragroup diversity is a further important consideration in planning care for ethnic elders. The black elderly are composed of three major groups: African Americans, African Caribbeans, and Africans, with the latter two groups demonstrating increasing immigration over the past 15 years (Baker, 1995). As a category, Native Americans represent well over 450 distinct tribes and nations. The Hispanic and Asian populations also have great intragroup diversity, with major variations in countries of origin and generation of immigration. For Hispanic elderly, about 50% are of Mexican origin; 15% Cuban; 12% Puerto Rican, and 25 % represent seven other countries of origin (Harper, 1995). Asian elderly represent the fastest growing group of ethnic elderly in the United States (Tanjasiri, Wallace, & Shibata, 1995). Currently about 30% of Asian elders are Chinese; 25% Japanese, 25% Filipino; 8% Korean; and 4% Vietnamese (U.S. Bureau of the Census, 1993); the Asian elders comprise more than 20 distinct ethnic groups who speak more than 30 different languages (Harada & Kim, 1995). For immigrants, there are considerable differences based on time residing in the United States, reasons for migration, prior social status and occupation, and acceptance or sponsorship by the host country.

Geographically, the configuration of ethnic elders becomes more complex. Elderly blacks, Asians, Native Americans, and Hispanics are concentrated in the West and the South. While elderly blacks are more dispersed than other groups, over half live in southern states. Asian elders are concentrated in western states (California, Hawaii, and Washington) and in New York. Further, specific population groups within these broader ethnic categories show even greater diversity. For example, among the Hispanic populations, a disproportionately greater number of Puerto Ricans reside in urban areas in the Northeast, Cubans in suburban areas in the Southeast, and Mexican Americans in rural areas of the Southwest (U.S. Bureau of the Census, 1993).

An additional important component regarding diversity among ethnic elderly concerns the nearly 8 million ethnic elderly of European descent, also called "white ethnic elderly." Although their ethnicity may not be as visible as that of the ethnic elderly of color, it remains just as salient a factor in planning and delivering nursing care. However, as a group, ethnic elderly of European descent remain the least studied and perhaps the least understood of all (Tripp-Reimer & Sorofman, 1988).

Clearly, the demographic data indicate that as a group, elders are now very heterogeneous and they are becoming more diverse. Yet this diversity has not received sufficient attention in the planning and delivery of health care.

HEALTH STATUS AND THE DISTRIBUTION OF CHRONIC ILLNESSES AMONG ETHNIC ELDERLY

Despite the last decade's general trends for healthier lifestyles and decreased morbidity rates for older persons, minority elders continue to demonstrate worse levels of health and well-being than their white counterparts. In general, members of ethnic groups tend to have shorter life expectancies than do members of the Anglo population. Blacks have an average life span that is about 5 years shorter than whites, and Native Americans, Eskimos, and Aleuts have the lowest life expectancy of all ethnic groups: at least 10 years below that of whites (U.S. Department of Health and Human Services, 1990). The 1985 Department of Health and Human Services Task Force identified causes of death that together account for more than 89% of the mortality observed among ethnic elderly that exceed that of Anglos: cancer, cardiovascular disease and stroke, chemical dependency, and diabetes. Further, mortality patterns also show striking differences among ethnic elderly for specific subtypes of diseases. For example, regarding patterns of cancer, the death rate for lung cancer is 45% higher for black males; esophageal cancer is three times higher for black men and women than whites; black women are 2.5 times more likely to die of cervical cancer; and the rates of mortality from stomach cancer and cancer of the uterus are higher for black elders than whites (Bazargan & Hamm-Baugh, 1995).

Chronic diseases are not randomly distributed within a population, but rather are associated with advanced age and socioeconomic status. In Western populations, an increase in life expectancy has led to an increase in the rate of chronic illnesses. Further, chronic disorders are not randomly distributed across ethnic groups. Summarizing recent research, Seccombe (1989) reports that elderly blacks, Hispanics, Koreans, Samoans, Guamanians, and Native Americans all have poorer health than do their white counterparts. Further, ethnic elderly also report higher rates of disability with over 25% having limited mobility as compared to only 17% of whites (Seccombe).

Elderly blacks are more likely than whites to be infirm and have chronic diseases. Blacks have the highest rates of cardiovascular disease in the world (Primas & Harper, 1991). Black elderly have more than twice the morbidity for hypertension and diabetes and are 50% more likely to have circulatory problems, arthritic diseases, and glaucoma (Johnson, Gibson, & Luckey, 1990; Willis, 1989). Chronic disorders have an earlier onset among blacks than whites, and they are more debilitating as they limit their activities to a greater extent (Bazargan & Hamm-Baugh, 1995; Ford, Haug, Jones, Roy, & Folmar, 1990). Black elders are more likely to be sick and disabled and to perceive themselves in poor health. They have higher rates of functional impairment and consistently demonstrate high rates of risk factors such as high blood pressure, obesity, increased use of alcohol and smoking (Fingerhut & Makuc, 1992; Harper & Alexander, 1990).

Among Hispanics, the leading causes of mortality are the same as in the general population: cardiovascular disease and cancer. However, rates of morbidity are higher among Hispanic elders. Other serious health problems that disproportionately affect Hispanic elderly include arthritis, cardiovascular disease, hypertension, cognitive impairment, depression, and cerebrovascular disease (National Institute on Aging, 1992). Diabetes is reported to be more than three times the general population. In particular, Hispanic elders also show higher limitations in activities of daily living and more days in bed a year due to illness than their white counterparts (Harper, 1995).

Native Americans are more than 10 times as likely to have diabetes than whites. For Native Americans, rates of diabetes, tuberculosis, hepatitis, and chronic dental problems far exceed the rates for whites (Manson & Brenneman, 1995). Diabetic complications are high among Native Americans, particularly nephropathy, end-stage renal disease, and lower-extremity amputation (Rousseau, 1995). Other key health problems include high rates of alcoholism and suicide. Several additional problems stem from high alcoholism and alcohol abuse, including cirrhosis of the liver and suicide (Harper, 1995). Despite poor quality of health statistics concerning Native American populations, the existing data depict a dire situation. The health status survey in 1986 found that 50% of Native American elders suffered from arthritis; over 16% were physically disabled; over half had significant hearing impairment (but less than 19% had hearing aids); and over 50%

had poor vision. Additionally, the survey determined that many health conditions were underreported to health providers. A final complicating factor is that there is a wide tribal variation in rates of chronic illness; for example, there are high rates of ischemic heart disease among Northern Plains tribes and low prevalence among Alaskan Natives and Native Americans in the Southwest.

For Asian Americans, the diversity of the population leads to greater intergroup differences in prevalence rates for many chronic illnesses. For example, diabetes is higher for Japanese than for other Asian groups; duodenal ulcer is higher in men from Vietnam, Cambodia, and Laos; gastric cancer is higher in native Hawaiians; and Filipinos demonstrate higher liver cancer rates. On the other hand, Japanese, Chinese, and Filipinos have lower rates of coronary artery disease (Douglas & Fujimoto, 1995). Other diseases that have higher prevalence among more recent immigrants and refugees from Asia include tuberculosis, hepatitis, and suicide (Primas & Harper, 1991).

Concerning chronic mental health problems, there is considerable ambiguity in the literature. Epidemiological research is very sparse regarding the differential distribution of mental disorders among ethnic elderly. The lack of comparable data makes generalizations regarding mental disorders and functioning among ethnic elders very difficult. However, the data that do exist suggest that African American elderly have relatively high rates of depression and severe cognitive impairment; Hispanic elder males have high rates of alcohol abuse, while Hispanic women have higher rates of affective disorders; Native Americans demonstrate increased rates of depression and alcohol abuse; and Asian Americans demonstrate higher rates of organic brain disorders (Jackson, Antonucci, & Gibson, 1995).

Multiple interacting risk factors contribute to these increased rates of chronic conditions among ethnic elderly. First, there may be genetic predisposition to certain types of chronic conditions such as diabetes, hypertension, or cancer. Second, cultural factors such as diet may be implicated as risk factors. However, of final and perhaps key importance is the relevance of socioeconomic factors. Chronic illnesses are known to accompany the poverty that is experienced by many ethnic elderly. Higher proportions of ethnic elderly live below the poverty level. For example, approximately 36% of black elderly fall below the federal poverty line as compared with 14% of elderly white Americans (U.S. Bureau of the Census, 1993). Wray (1992) noted that given their generally lower socioeconomic status, it is not surprising that ethnic elderly have a higher prevalence of chronic disorders and disabling conditions than do elderly whites. Ethnic differences in health states begin early in life and continue into old age (Seccombe, 1989).

A second category of factors that contribute to the increased disability experienced by ethnic elderly with chronic disorders concerns access as well as diagnostic and treatment factors related to biomedical health care. One reason for this variation is that many diagnostic indicators of chronic disease are not detectable if persons do not seek routine health care. Consequently, many chronic disorders may be underreported among ethnic populations with low rates of access to and utilization of health care.

Second, if health care is sought, there may be considerable diagnostic biases that warrant attention; the higher prevalence rates of chronic impairments may stem from atypical disease presentation or from diagnostic or testing errors. Hypertension has unique characteristics in African Americans as a whole. It tends to appear at an earlier age, is generally more severe, and is associated with higher rates of morbidity and mortality. Blacks have a more severe salt sensitivity, with low plasma rennin levels and a tendency toward volume expansion. Treatment modalities may differ, with beta-blockers often being less effective in controlling hypertension (Brangman, 1995). Testing issues in diagnosis also are relevant issues with ethnic elderly. Because the Mini-Mental State Examination (MMSE) scores tend to correlate with social status and educational level, one reason for low MMSE scores among African Americans is their relatively lower levels of education. However, other research indicates that the higher rates of cognitive impairment result from higher rates of multi-infarct dementia due to higher incidence of hypertension in the African American population (Baker, 1988). Finally, there is evidence to indicate that there may be possible diagnostic biases attributable to cultural differences between patients and practitioners. For example, research indicates that blacks tend to be overdiagnosed with schizophrenia and underdiagnosed with depression. Further, Cohen (1993) reports that older low-income black patients with altered affect and thought content characteristic of schizophrenia are more often misdiagnosed as having Alzheimer's Disease than their white counterparts.

Third, practitioner variations in treatment plans also play a part in the disability experienced by ethnic elders. For example, even when blacks gain access to the health care system, they are less likely than whites to receive certain surgical or other therapies. Black men are only half as likely as whites to undergo angiography and twice as likely to undergo bypass surgery after myocardial infarction (MI). There are also racial disparities with regard to long-term dialysis and organ (kidney) transplant. Recent statistics show blacks account for 33% of persons with end-stage renal disease, but only 21% of renal transplant patients (Council on Ethical and Judicial Affairs, 1990).

Finally, the medications used to treat ethnic elders may have different pharmacologic effects due to genetic polymorphisms that affect the metabolism of the medication. For example, common antihypertensive medications (including beta-blockers, diuretics calcium channel antagonists, and angiotensin converting enzyme (ACE) inhibitors produce different clinical responses in black, Chinese, and Caucasian elders. While black elders tend to respond better to diuretics than to beta-blocking agents, the Chinese are considerably more sensitive than Caucasians to the effects of beta-blockers on heart rate and blood pressure (Levy, 1993). Unfortunately, far too little knowledge regarding ethnic variation in pharmacokinetics is available and that which is available has not been disseminated widely to health professionals.

DEFINING AND EVALUATING CHRONIC DISORDERS

Elders in all ethnic groups experience chronic conditions in their later years. However, one's ethnic affiliation strongly influences the definition, recognition, and evaluation of chronic conditions. There is a potential for disparity between an individual's subjective perception of his or her health state and that of a biomedical practitioner. Individuals may define themselves as "healthy" even in the presence of obvious pathology. Many conditions are perceived as "normal" because of their high frequency in a population. The definition of health "need" among elders has been demonstrated to vary with ethnicity (Cox, 1986). At other times, illness is not acknowledged because it is considered to be merely a normal and unavoidable part of aging. There is a considerable propensity for elders to attribute their symptoms to the effects of age, rather than to an illness (Keller, Leventhal, Prohaska, & Leventhal, 1989). Harper (1995) points out that many physiological changes such as edema, stiffness, dizziness, constipation, and urinary urgency may be viewed as unavoidable. For example, Saravanabhavan and Marshall (1994) point out that elderly Native Americans tend to accept ill health as a part of their old age, and Brangman (1995) notes that many elderly blacks do not define a condition as an illness unless it interferes with their functioning.

A corollary issue in elders' definition of their condition is that the condition may be undetected. Any chronic conditions such as hypertension, diabetes, and renal or respiratory problems may not show strong symptoms that are recognizable by lay persons. These "hidden" diseases are detectable by laboratory tests or with specialized equipment. Often, chronic illnesses are not identified because they are not detected. For multiple and complex reasons, ethnic elders often do not received regular health screenings. As a result, chronic conditions often are not recognized in their early stages (Harper & Alexander, 1990). Lack of detection may be attributable to issues of access, but fear also plays a role. Matthews, Lannin, and Mitchell (1994) found that black women with breast cancer often had delayed mammographies even when they sensed they may have had a problem with the rationale that refusing to acknowledge the problem is somehow protective from suffering the full effect of the cancer. Similarly, Hmong immigrants often believe that discussing a potential health problem before it occurs increases its likelihood (Boult & Boult, 1995).

A third reason that chronic disorders may not come to the attention of health practitioners is that the condition is stigmatized by the ethnic group and the sufferer resists disclosure of information that could bring both individual and family shame. For example, Mexican American males often view emotional problems as signs of a weak character (Cheung & Snowden, 1990). Korean elderly were found less likely to identify elder abuse or to seek treatment for it when compared with black and Caucasian elders (Moon & Williams, 1993); the issue of "family shame" was often cited in the rationale for nonidentification. The issue of stigmatized problems may be seen for many chronic mental disorders, especially for elders of Asian and Hispanic descent.

A final reason that chronic disorders are not so identified by ethnic elders may be the result of a lay health system that explains illness and defines appropriate treatments and healers. However, this lay system may rest outside, or overlap with, that of biomedicine. The topic "Ethnic Models of Sickness and Treatment" is explored next in detail.

ETHNIC MODELS OF SICKNESS AND TREATMENT

All ethnic groups have indigenous health care systems that include methods of prevention, diagnosis, and treatment of health problems as they are diagnosed by and for members of that group. Lay systems of treatment include care by self, family, lay healers (such as herbalists), or indigenous specialists (such as Native American medicine men, Mexican American *curanderas,* or African American root doctors). Indigenous health systems are often highly complex, interrelated dimensions that profoundly affect the trajectory of chronic illness for ethnic elderly.

One of the most common examples of an indigenous health care system is that found in East Asia. This system, which has roots in China, holds that illness results when the body's equilibrium is disrupted. The distal cause of an illness may be natural, supernatural, or humoral forces (Lum, 1995). Health (physical, psychological, and social) is based on a balance of complimentary *yin* and *yang* forces in combination with vital energy (*chi*). An excess in *yang* causes symptoms such as constipation, fevers, and sore throats. Examples of deficiency states that are considered to be *yin* conditions are diarrhea, dizziness, and indigestion, Each category of symptoms (*yin* or *yang*) is treated by the principle of opposition. *Yang* treatments are used for *yin* states; *yin* treatments for *yang* states. Examples of hot or *yang* treatments include foods rich in fats or proteins, or highly spiced foods. Antibiotics and most Western prescription medications are also considered *yang* treatments. *Yin* or cold treatments include acupuncture, many herbal teas, and fruits and vegetables (Tripp-Reimer, Johnson, & Rios, 1994). Chinese elders in the United States may prefer the services of herbalists and "Chinese doctors" rather than those of a biomedically trained physician (Yeo, 1991). However, even more commonly, they prefer to use recommended herbal remedies rather than seeking consultation from a traditional specialist. When treatments recommended by biomedical practitioners are used, they may be modified. For example, taking half a prescribed dose is a common practice among Chinese elders; this practice is based on the belief that Western doses are too strong ("hot") for them (Yeo).

Traditional Korean medicine represents one of the many derivations of the Chinese system. In states of health, there is a balance among the complimentary forces (*um* and *yang*) in combination with vital energy (*ki*). Illness is caused by imbalance in the physical, spiritual, or social realms. Treatment may occur in the home or in a *hanbang,* a traditional Korean medical clinic. In the *hanbang,* possible treatments include *ch'im* (acupuncture), *hanyak* (traditional herbal remedies), *d'um* (moxibustion), and *buhwang* (cupping). Traditional Korean clinics and physicians (*hanui*) are most often visited by more recent and elder Korean immigrants (Pang, 1989).

Traditional modes of therapy are particularly sought when an illness is considered to be a folk illness. For example, *hwabyung* is a folk illness caused from stress and oppressive relations that result in unexpressed anger. Symptoms of *hwabyung* include elements of both depression and somatic illnesses (Pang, 1990). Traditional healers may be viewed as most appropriate when this is the lay diagnosis, because the traditional healer is expected to offer treatments that will bring the physical, spiritual, and social realms into balance.

A second major group of traditions are those based in Mexico, the Carribean, and Central and South America. This cluster is a set of systems based in the syntheses of traditions stemming from indigenous (native) peoples, African slaves, and Spanish, Portuguese, and French colonialists. The original indigenous system is most apparent in use of local herbs and tonics for treatments. The colonialist influence is based in the Hippocratic model of pathology that Europeans brought to the New World in the 16th and 17th centuries. According to this model (and similar to that of the Chinese), illness is largely due to imbalance. A disproportion of hot or cold will lead to illness. Cold illnesses are often caused by an intrusion of cold into the body through drafts or winds (termed *mal aire*), which weaken the body and increase susceptibility to illnesses. An excess of heat is generally within the body itself. Symptoms indicative of "cold" include chest pain and abdominal pain; whereas, symptoms indicative of a "hot" state include fever, rashes, and renal problems. Foods and herbs are also classified into hot and cold categories, and like the Chinese system, the treatment is by the principle of opposition. "Hot" foods and herbs treat "cold illnesses" and vice versa. The colonialists also imposed Catholicism, which included the belief in *castigo,* or illness being caused as punishment for sins. African slaves brought a religious tradition based on a pantheon of gods and deities. The co-occurrence of these systems evolved into the numerous syncretic religious/healing systems found today, including *Curanderismo* (Mexico), *Espiritismo* (Puerto Rico), *Vodun* (Haiti), *Shango* (Trinidad), and *Macumba* and *Umbanda* (Brazil) (Tripp-Reimer, 1992).

The indigenous system of many African Americans includes beliefs in both natural and unnatural categories. Natural illnesses occur from lack of moderation or exposure to air (especially cold) or impurities in air, water, or food. Impurities can accumulate in the body and result in illness; there is considerable concern with maintaining normal body functions, including bowel elimination, blood flow (and general blood condition), and menstrual regularity. Natural illnesses also include those sent by God either as punishment or as a test of faith. Unnatural illnesses result from the work of evil forces, including the devil, or witchcraft worked through a "hex" or "fix." Treatments for unnatural illnesses are based in religious healing, countermagic, or additional protections (crosses, charms, asafetida bags) (Brangman, 1995; Gregg & Curry, 1994; Snow, 1974, 1993).

Folk remedies are often a key element within traditional medical systems. Further, their use may be retained even after traditional specialists are no longer available in an ethnic community. However, some ethnic elders demonstrate a definite "shift" toward use of over-the-counter (OTC) remedies. In part, this shift results from decreased availability of herbs and increased availability and ease of preparation of OTCs. For example, Czech elders reported a prior high use of a mixture of goose grease and turpentine as a chest liniment for colds, they now report use of Vics Vaporub (Tripp-Reimer & Sorofman, 1989). Use of home remedies and conditions most commonly treated also vary by ethnic groups. Chinese elders in San Francisco are reported to rely more on herbal remedies for indigestion, whereas blacks and Mexican Americans tend to use laxatives to cleanse the gastrointestinal track (Boyd, Shimp, & Hackney, 1984; Hess, 1986). In all cases, however, it is incumbent on nurses to identify the pharmacologic properties of the remedies. While many remedies are beneficial for their intended purpose, others may be harmful (inherently, or in combination with other medications). For example, use of mercury as a therapy is widespread among Puerto Rican and Mexican American elderly. Mercury is used for good luck and to protect a person from the envy of others (Zayas & Ozuah, 1996). Among Asian elderly, ginseng is commonly used to retain vitality; however, it may also have antihypertensive effects that may overpower or counteract other medications. Further, many herbal drugs used by Asian elders have anticholinergic properties that make the elders more susceptible to acute confusion (delirium) (Douglas & Fujimoto, 1995). Home remedies commonly used by African Americans also may have considerable health risks. For example, sassafras root bark contains a hepatotoxic agent, and sulfur (used to treat dyspnea) can induce metabolic acidosis (Boyd et al.). Thus while folk remedies may be an important part of elder's self-care practices, their use—alone or in combination with other OTC or prescribed medicines—warrants evaluation.

Traditional medical systems provide explanations for and treatments of illness that are culturally familiar to ethnic elders. However, their degree of use may vary depending on multiple interacting factors, including the elder's generation of immigration, access to traditional and scientific practitioners, level of education, gender, and English language proficiency.

The importance of multiple and varied understandings within traditional health systems can be illustrated in the following example of a common chronic illness: hypertension. Interviewing Hispanic immigrants, Ailinger (1988) found that over one-half believed that hypertension was caused or aggravated by *cólera* (anger), *susto* (fright), living at a high altitude, and too much blood in the system. Treatments used included changing climate, eating bananas and pears, drinking chamomile tea, and also drinking ice water. In contrast, Garro (1988) found that Ojibwa considered hypertension a "white man's illness" and therefore not amenable to treatment by Indian healers. The Ojibwa attributed hypertension to too much worry, alcohol, and overexertion. In Detroit, Bailey (1991) found multiple lay specialists (herbalists, magic store vendors) being used for hypertension treatments, with remedies including Epsom salts, garlic tablets, vinegar, lemon tea, dandelion and valerian root. In a similar vein, persons from the West Indies identified stress or worry as a cause of their hypertension. Although all identified the importance of controlling blood pressure, less than half were compliant with prescribed regimens. Most West Indians regularly "left off" drug treatments for a few days or weeks. The West Indian rationales for "leaving off" were the danger of mixing hypertensive drugs with alcohol, the harmful effects of the drugs themselves, and the possibility of being addicted to the drugs. While they were not taking their regularly prescribed medications, West Indians often used alternative medicines, including blood tonics, herbal teas, and bitters (Morgan & Watkins, 1988).

FORMAL AND INFORMAL CARE

Ethnic elderly tend to use informal support structures more than Caucasians (Gibson, 1989). These informal support structures take the form of family, friendship networks, and religious affiliates. It is important to note substantial cultural variations in attitudes toward care of the elderly, in the identification and recruitment of care providers, and in normative patterns of behavior for the persons who assist chronically ill elderly.

Although particular features vary among different ethnic groups, the concept of family is universal. Further, for every ethnic group, the family generally constitutes the most important support system for the elder. This is often most evident when chronic illness or frailty is most pronounced. Families may be viewed as primarily lineal or collateral in form (Tripp-Reimer,

Johnson, & Rios, 1994; White-Means & Thornton, 1990). In lineal families, the most significant relationships are between spouses and between parents and children. Examples of lineal families include most Asian family systems (Chinese, Japanese, Korean) and most northern European (English, German, Norwegian). Collateral-oriented families extend the informal care system to siblings, extended kin networks, and friends. Commonly, collateral-based families can be found among African Americans and southern and eastern Europeans (including Italians, Hispanics, and Polish).

Clarke and Neidert (1992) examined patterns of living with relatives among American elderly of European origin. In general, they reported that elders of southern or eastern European backgrounds were more likely to reside with relatives than were their northwestern European counterparts. Further, they found no decrease in this pattern as generational depth increased in the United States. These findings support earlier work reporting that in contrast to Czech and Norwegian families, Greek elders and their adult children tended to prefer coresidence, particularly if the Greek elder was frail (Tripp-Reimer, 1992).

There is considerable information concerning informal support structures and patterns among the elderly in major ethnic categories in the United States. However, intragroup variation remains a key consideration. For example, Hispanic elders are more likely than either black or Caucasian elders to share housing and receive help from an adult child (Lubben & Becerra, 1987). However, within the larger cluster "Hispanic," considerable differences are apparent: Cubans tend to rely on children and friends in their neighborhood; Mexican Americans tend to rely on extended family networks; and Puerto Ricans appear to be the least reliant on informal support systems (Angel & Angel, 1992; Angel & Hogan, 1992; Mangum, Garcia, Kosberg, Mullins & Barresi, 1994).

While the size of the total caregiver network to older blacks does not differ from Caucasians, the kinds of informal support vary considerably (Burton et al., 1995). Although black families strongly endorse family support for the elderly, blacks tend to have a more diverse group of caregivers, including more extended family members and close friends than do other ethnic groups (Baker, 1995; Cox, 1993; Gibson, 1986; Ulbrich & Bradsher, 1993; Ulbrich & Warheit, 1989). Black families tend to expand network membership in two directions: by mobilizing relatives on the periphery of kinship networks (e.g., cousins, nieces, nephews) and by extending kinship networks through fictive kin (Johnson & Barer, 1990). Further, support from friends was more important than from close family members in reducing the onset of depression in chronically ill black elders (Barzargan & Hamm-Baugh, 1995). However, a considerable subset of black elders (nearly 20%) were found to have no weekly contact with any friend or relative (Johnson & Barer, 1990); the majority of members of this subset had serious mental or physical illness, including chronic pulmonary disease with continuous use of oxygen, high incidence of schizophrenia, depression, alcoholism, and dementia. Further, older black men seem most isolated when visits or phone calls are considered (Spitze & Miner, 1992).

Further, there appear to be differences in the amount of caregiving provided by informal networks. Black caregivers perform more caregiving activities and care for persons with greater functional and cognitive impairment despite the fact that they report less burden (Fredman, Daly, & Lazur, 1995) and role strain (Mui, 1992).

Asian societies are characterized by an ethnic of filial piety that stems from Confucian teachings termed *Hyo* in Korean, *Hsiao* in Chinese, and *Ko* in Japanese (Sung, 1990). Main precepts of filial piety include respecting one's parents, bringing no dishonor to parents or other family members, and taking good care of parents as they become frail (Sung, 1995). In the East, this care is generally the responsibility of the eldest son (and his wife); however, in the United States, the pattern of caregiving is shifting more responsibility to daughters (Choi, 1993; Tran, 1991). When chronic illness evolves to greater levels of disability, there is a greater likelihood that elders will be cared for by children, this is particularly true for elders who migrated after 1965 (Burr & Mutchler, 1993).

HEALTH SERVICES UTILIZATION BY ETHNIC ELDERS

Ethnic elders are underserved throughout the continuum of care for acute long-term care settings for both physical and mental health problems. These rates of underutilization stand in striking contrast to their documented need for such services. Ethnic elders are often stereotyped as traditionalists who are unwilling to participate in mainstream health programs. This inappropriate characterization has been termed the "cultural aversion hypothesis" (Morrison, 1982). The assumption of health and social service providers that ethnic elders do not prefer to use the continuum of health services available is often erroneous and places undue burden on elders and their informal networks. Issues with each of the four main components of access

— (a) availability, (b) affordability, (c) accessibility, and (d) acceptability— continue to block or inhibit ethnic elders' full participation in the formal health care continuum.

Although ethnic elders may use emergency rooms (ER) as a source of primary care at higher rates than Caucasians (Damron-Rodriguez, Wallace, & Kington, 1994; Wolinsky et al., 1989), they often do not have access to discretionary preventive and treatment services that would allow early diagnosis and consistent treatment of chronic conditions (Wolinsky, Callahan, Fitzgerald, & Johnson, 1992). This pattern often precludes elders from obtaining consistent primary care for their complex chronic health problems. Overall, physician use varies by ethnicity. Asian and Pacific elders seek primary care at less than half the rate of Caucasian elderly, despite a high rate of need. Multiple factors have been implicated in the underutilization of primary health providers, including high physician turnover leading to lack of consistent provider, lack of insurance coverage or inability to cover copayments, transportation, difficulties with translation (or need to repeatedly recite medical history to new provider), fragmentation of services, and depersonalization (Boult & Boult, 1995; Damon-Rodriguez et al., 1994; Mui & Burnette, 1994; Petchers & Milligan, 1988; Snowden & Cheung, 1990; Tanjasiri et al., 1995; Wolinsky et al., 1989; Wykle & Kaskel, 1991).

The pattern of ethnic elders to underutilize formal or professional services is consistent across the continuum of care and has been demonstrated for community-based and in-home long-term care health and social services (Damron-Rodriguez et al., 1994; Miner, 1995; Mitchell, 1995; Wallace, 1995).

The issues involved in underutilization of services differ dramatically across ethnic groups. This point will be illustrated by highlighting some of the issues for distinct groups of ethnic elders. Native American elders are generally covered under the service provision of the Indian Health Services (IHS), which has a statutory responsibility to meet the health needs of American Indians. However, because the IHS tends to define its mission in terms of acute care, the rapidly increasing long-term care needs of the growing numbers of aging tribal members are largely ignored. John (1991) points out that a key issue problem confronting tribal elders is a policy of age discrimination in resource allocation within the Indian Health Service. Specifically, he notes that the IHS concentrates its resources on the health problems of younger tribal members through the Resource Allocation Method, which is based on the calculation of the Years of Productive Life

Lost. This strategy virtually ignores health issues for elders over age 65. For example, in 1989, there were only 10 reservation-based nursing homes that housed 435 residents (Manson, 1989a); in 1995, there were only 15 such facilities (Rousseau, 1995). As a result, placement in a nursing home may be distressing to tribal elders because the facilities may be located at a great distance from kin precluding frequent visits, language barriers commonly exist between tribal elders and nonnative caregivers, and nursing home customs and diets may be unfamiliar (Rousseau, 1995; Shomaker, 1990). Further, there are also very few community-based home services that could aid families, despite the estimation that at least 46% of older tribal members are assisted by extended family members to accomplish activities of daily living (Manson, 1989b).

Hispanic elderly have demonstrated for at least 20 years their underutilization of nursing home care. Currently, Mexican American data indicate that they use nursing home services half as often as non-Hispanic white elders. Further, Hispanic elders residing in nursing homes have been found to be significantly more disabled than their non-Hispanic counterparts. While there is a dramatic lack of research regarding reasons for these patterns, common reasons invoked include care that is culturally inappropriate, inaccessibility to family, inability to pay for services, and cultural bias against institutionalization (Chiodo, Kanten, Gerety, Mulrow, & Cornell, 1994; National Institute on Aging, 1992).

Black elders do not demonstrate high use of community-based long-term care programs (only about 12% report using a senior center) (Kart, 1991). Similarly, they are underrepresented in nursing homes. At comparable rates of frailty, the likelihood of nursing home admissions for blacks is less than half that of whites (Belgrave & Bradsher, 1994; Belgrave, Wykle, & Choi, 1993; Greene & Ondrich, 1990). In a study of poor urban dwellers in Ohio, Groger (1994) reported that elderly blacks tended to enter a nursing home only after they defined themselves as incompetent, had limited social support, had current helpers unable to increase their efforts, and were unable to mobilize additional helpers. However, for long-term care admissions, the issue of frank racial discrimination is now receiving more attention as a primary barrier. In a dramatic study of race as a barrier to long-term institutional care in North Carolina, Falcone and Broyles (1994) found that nursing homes demonstrate "inescapable" evidence of discrimination on the basis of race in admitting patients. Their study used data from nearly 3,000 patients in 76 hospitals who were awaiting placement in long-term care facilities, and it controlled for most variables often employed to explain underutilization: patients' payment source for long-term care for their chronic conditions or special care requirements, demographic characteristics, family cooperativeness, and multiple other factors. Thus poverty, geographical isolation, and discrimination are increasingly seen as primary reasons rather than the prior characterization that relied most heavily on personal preference.

It seems apparent that multiple factors need to be addressed in considering service utilization by ethnic elders. Current barriers have been well summarized as (1) knowledge barriers (awareness of need for and existence of services), (2) access barriers (physical, geographic, financial, and linguistic access), and (3) intent barriers (discrimination from providers and preferences by participants) (Yeatts, Crow, & Folts, 1992). Nursing can and should play a key role in reducing barriers and increasing formal service participation by ethnic elders.

REFERENCES

Ailinger, R. L. (1988). Folk beliefs about high blood pressure in Hispanic immigrants. *Western Journal of Nursing Research, 10*, 629–636.

Angel, J. L., & Angel, R. J. (1992). Age at migration, social connection, and well-being among elderly Hispanics. *Journal of Aging and Health, 4,* 480–499.

Angel, J. L., & Hogan, D. P. (1992). The demography of minority aging populations. *Journal of Family History, 17*(1), 95–115.

Bailey, E. J. (1991). Hypertension: An analysis of Detroit African American health care treatment patterns. *Human Organizations, 50*(3), 287–296.

Baker, F. M. (1988). Dementing illness and black Americans. In J. S. Jackson, P. Newton, A. Ostfield, D. Savage, & E. Schneider (Eds.), *The black American elderly: Research on physical and psychosocial health* (pp. 215–233). New York: Springer.

Baker, F. M. (1995). Mental health issues in elderly African Americans. *Clinics in Geriatric Medicine, 11*(1), 1–14.

Bazargan, M., & Hamm-Baugh, B. P. (1995). The relationship between chronic illness and depression in a community of urban black elderly persons. *Journal of Gerontology: Social Sciences, 50B,* S119–S127.

Belgrave, L. L., & Bradsher, J. E. (1994). Health as a factor in institutionalization: Disparities between African Americans and whites. *Research on Aging, 16*(2), 115–141.

Belgrave, L. L., Wykle, M. L., & Choi, J. M. (1993). Health, double jeopardy, and culture: The use of institutionalization by African-Americans. *Gerontologist, 33*(3), 379–385.

Boult, L., & Boult, C. (1995). Underuse of physician services by older Asian-Americans. *Journal of the American Geriatrics Society, 43,* 408–411.

Boyd, E. L., Shimp, L. A., & Hackney, M. J. (1984). *Home remedies and the black elderly: A reference manual for health care providers.* Ann Arbor: University of Michigan.

Brangman, S. A. (1995). African-American elders: Implications for health care providers. *Clinics in Geriatric Medicine, 111*(1), 15–24.

Burr, J. A., & Mutchler, J. E. (1993). Nativity, acculturation, and economic status: Explanations of Asian American living arrangements in later life. *Journal of Gerontology: Social Sciences, 48*(2), S55–S63.

Burton, L., Kasper, J., Shore, A., Cagney, K., LaVeist, T., Cubbin, C. & German, P. (1995). The structure of informal care: Are there differences by race? *Gerontologist, 35*(6), 744–752.

Cheung, F. K., & Snowden, L. R. (1990). Community mental health and ethnic minority populations. *Community Mental Health Journal, 20,* 277–291.

Chiodo, L. K., Kanten, D. N., Gerety, M. B., Mulrow, C. D., & Cornell, J. E. (1994). Functional status of Mexican American nursing home residents. *Journal of the American Geriatrics Society, 42,* 293–296.

Choi, H. (1993). Cultural and noncultural factors as determinants of caregiver burden for the impaired elderly in South Korea. *Gerontologist, 33,* 8–15.

Clarke, C. J., & Neidert, L. J. (1992). Living arrangement of the elderly: An examination of differences according to ancestry and generation. *Gerontologist, 32,* 796–804.

Cohen, G. D. (1993). African American issues in geriatric psychiatry: A perspective on research opportunities. *Journal of Geriatric Psychiatry and Neurology, 6,* 195–199.

Council on Ethical and Judicial Affairs. (1990). Black-white disparities in health care. *JAMA, 263,* 2344–2347.

Cox, C. (1986). Physician utilization by three groups of ethnic elderly. *Medical Care, 24,* 667–676.

Cox, C. (1993). Service needs and interests: A comparison of African American and white caregivers seeking Alzheimer assistance. *American Journal of Alzheimer's Care and Related Disorders and Research, 8*(3), 33–40.

Damron-Rodriguez, J., Wallace, S., & Kington, R. (1994). Service utilization and minority elders: Appropriateness, accessibility and acceptability. In D. Padgett (Ed.), *Handbook on ethnicity, aging and mental health* (pp. 45–63). London: Greenwood.

Douglas, K. C., & Fujimoto, D. (1995). Asian Pacific elders: Implications for health care providers. *Clinics in Geriatric Medicine, 111*(1), 69–82.

Falcone, D., & Broyles, R. (1994). Access to long-term care: Race as a barrier. *Journal of Health Politics, Policy, and Law, 19*(3), 583–595.

Fingerhut, L. A., & Makuc, D. M. (1992). Mortality among minority populations in the United States. *American Journal of Public Health, 82,* 1168–1170.

Ford, A. B., Haug, M. R., Jones, P. K., Roy, A. W., & Folmar, S. J. (1990). Race-related differences among elderly urban residents: A cohort study, 1975–1984. *Journal of Gerontology: Social Sciences, 45*(4), S163–S171.

Fredman, L., Daly, M. P., & Lazur, A. M. (1995). Burden among white and black caregivers to elderly adults. *Journal of Gerontology: Social Sciences, 50B,* S110–S118.

Garro, L. (1988). Explaining high blood pressure: Variation in knowledge about illness. *American Ethnologist, 15*(1), 98–119.

Gibson, R. C. (1986). Older black Americans. *Generations (SU),* 35–39.

Gibson, R. C. (1989). Minority aging research: Opportunity and challenge. *Journal of Gerontology, 44*(1), 52–53.

Greene, V. L., & Ondrich, J. I. (1990). Risk factors for nursing home admissions and exits: A discrete-time hazard function approach. *Journal of Gerontology, 45*(6), S250–S258.

Gregg, J., & Curry, R. H. (1994). Explanatory models for cancer among African-American women at two Atlanta neighborhood health centers: The importance for a cancer screening program. *Social Science and Medicine, 39,* 519–526.

Groger, L. (1994). Limit of support and reaction to illness: An exploration of black elders' pathways to long-term care settings. *Journal of Cross-Cultural Gerontology, 9,* 369–387.

Harada, N. D., & Kim, L. S. (1995). Use of mental health services by older Asian and Pacific Islander Americans. In D. Padgett (Ed.), *Handbook on ethnicity, aging, and mental health* (pp. 185–202). London: Greenwood.

Harper, M. S. (1995). Caring for the special needs of aging minorities. *Health Care Trends and Transitions, 6*(4), 8–20.

Harper, M. S., & Alexander, C. D. (1990). *Profile of the black elderly. Minority aging: Essential curricula content for selected health and allied health professors* (No. HRS-8-DV90-4). Rockville, MD: USDHHS: HRSA.

Hess, P. (1986). Chinese and Hispanic elders and OTC drugs. *Geriatric Nursing, 7*(6), 314–318.

Jackson, J. S., Antonucci, T. C., & Gibson, R. C. (1995). Ethnic and cultural factors in research on aging and mental health: A life-course perspective. In D. Padgett (Ed.), *Handbook on ethnicity, aging and mental health* (pp. 21–46). London: Greenwood.

John, R. (1991). The state of research on American Indian elders' health, income security, and social support networks. In *Minority elders: Longevity, economics and health* (pp. 38–50). Washington, DC: Gerontological Society of America.

Johnson, C. L., & Barer, B. M. (1990). Families and networks among older inner-city blacks. *Gerontologist, 30,* 726–733.

Johnson, H. R., Gibson, R. C., & Luckey, I. (1990). Health and social characteristics: Implications for services. In Z. Harel, E. McKinney, & M. William (Eds.), *Black aged: Understanding diversity and service needs* (pp. 69–81). Newbury Park, CA: Sage.

Kart, C. S. (1991). Variation in long-term care service use by aged blacks. *Journal of Aging and Health, 3*(4), 511–526.

Keller, M., Leventhal, H., Prohaska, T., & Leventhal, E. (1989). Beliefs about aging and illness in a community sample. *Research in Nursing and Health, 12,* 247–255.

Levy, R. A. (1993). Ethnic and racial differences in response to medicines: Preserving individualized therapy in managed pharmaceutical programs. *Pharmaceutical Medicine, 7,* 139–165.

Lubben, J. E., & Becerra, R. M. (1987). Social support among Black, Mexican and Chinese elderly. In D. E. Gelfand & C. M. Barresi (Eds.), *Ethical dimensions of aging* (pp. 130–144). New York: Springer.

Lum, O. M. (1995). Health status of Asians and Pacific Islanders. *Clinics in Geriatric Medicine, 111*(1), 53–68.

Mangum, W. O, Garcia, J. L, Kosberg, J. I., Mullins, L. C., & Barresi, C. M. (1994). Racial/ethnic variations in informal caregiving. *Educational Gerontology, 20,* 715–731.

Manson, S. M. (1989a). Long-term care in American Indian communities: Issues for planning and research. *Gerontologist, 29*(1), 38–44.

Manson, S. M. (1989b). Provider assumptions about long-term care in American Indian communities. *Gerontologist, 29*(3), 355–358.

Manson, S. M., & Brenneman, D. L. (1995). Chronic disease among older American Indians: Preventing depressive symptoms and related problems of coping. In D. Padgett (Ed.), *Handbook on ethnicity, aging, and mental health* (pp. 389–403). London: Greenwood.

Matthews, H. F., Lannin, D. R., & Mitchell, J. P. (1994). Coming to terms with advanced breast cancer: Black women's narratives from eastern North Carolina. *Social Science and Medicine, 38*(6), 789–800.

Miner, S. (1995). Racial differences in family support and formal service utilization among older persons: A nonrecursive model. *Journal of Gerontology: Social Sciences, 50B*(3), S143–S153.

Mitchell, J. (1995). Service awareness and use among older North Carolinians. *Journal of Applied Gerontology, 14*(2), 193–209.

Moon, A., & Williams, O. (1993). Perceptions of elder abuse and help-seeking patterns among African-American, Caucasian American, and Korean-American elderly women. *Gerontologist, 33*(3), 386–395.

Morgan, M., & Watkins, C. J. (1988). Managing hypertension: Beliefs and responses to medication among cultural groups. *Sociology of Health and Illness, 10,* 561–578.

Morrison, B. (1982). Sociocultural dimensions: Nursing homes and the minority aged. *Journal of Gerontological Social Work, 5,* 127–145.

Mui, A. (1992). Caregiver strain among black and white daughter caregivers: A role theory perspective. *Gerontologist, 32,* 203–212.

Mui, A. C., & Burnette, D. (1994). Long-term care service use by frail elders: Is ethnicity a factor? *Gerontologist, 34*(2), 190–198.

National Institute on Aging. (1992). *Hispanic aging: Issues in research and communication.*

Pang, K. Y. (1989). The practice of traditional Korean medicine in Washington, DC. *Social Science and Medicine, 28,* 875–884.

Pang, K. Y. (1990). Hwabyung: The construction of a Korean popular illness among Korean elderly immigrant women in the United States. *Culture, Medicine, and Psychiatry, 14,* 495–512.

Petchers, M. K., & Milligan, S. E. (1988). Access to health care in a black urban elderly population. *Gerontologist, 28,* 213–217.

Primas, M. E., & Harper, M. S. (1991). Psychosocial care for racial and ethnic minority elderly. In M. Hayes (Ed.), *Management and care of the elderly.* Newbury Park, CA: Sage.

Rousseau, P. (1995). Native-American elders: Health care status. *Clinics in Geriatric Medicine, 111*(1), 83–98.

Saravanabhavan, R. C., & Marshall, C. A. (1994). The older Native American Indian with disabilities: Implications for providers of health care and human services. *Journal of Multicultural Counseling and Development, 22,* 182–194.

Seccombe, K. (1989). Ethnicity or socioeconomic status? Health differences between elder Alaska Natives and whites. *Gerontologist, 29*(4), 551–556.

Shomaker, D. (1990). Health care, cultural expectations, and frail elderly Navajo grandmothers. *Journal of Cross-Cultural Gerontology, 5,* 21–34.

Snow, L. F. (1974). Folk medical beliefs and their implications for care of patients. *Annals of Internal Medicine, 81,* 82–96.

Snow, L. F. (1993). *Walkin' over medicine.* Boulder, CO: Westview Press.

Snowden, L. R., & Cheung, F. K. (1990). Use of inpatient mental health services by members of ethnic minority groups. *American Psychologist, 45*(3), 347–355.

Spitze, G., & Miner, S. (1992). Gender differences in adult child contact among black elderly parents. *Gerontologist, 32,* 213–218.

Sung, K. (1995). Measures and dimensions of filial piety in Korea. *Gerontologist, 35*(2), 240–247.

Sung, T. (1990). A new look at filial piety: Ideals and practices of family-centered parent care in Korea. *Gerontologist, 30,* 610–617.

Tanjasiri, S. P., Wallace, S. P., & Shibata, K. (1995). Picture imperfect: Hidden problems among Asian Pacific Islander elderly. *Gerontologist, 35(6),* 735–760.

Tran, T. V. (1991). Family living arrangement and social adjustment among three ethnic groups of elderly Indochinese refugees. *International Journal of Aging and Human Development, 32,* 91–102.

Tripp-Reimer, T. (1992). Cultural assessment. In J. Bellach & B. Edlund (Eds.), *Nursing assessment and diagnosis* (pp. 208–231). Boston: Jones and Bartlett Publishers.

Tripp-Reimer, T., Johnson, R., & Rios, H. (1994). Cultural dimensions in gerontological nursing. In M. Stanley & P. G. Beare (Eds.), *Gerontological nursing* (pp. 28–36). Philadelphia: J. B. Lippincott.

Tripp-Reimer, T., & Lauer, G. (1987). Ethnicity and families with chronic illness. In L. Wright & M. Leahey (Eds.), *Families and chronic illness* (pp. 77–100). Philadelphia: Springhouse Corporation.

Tripp-Reimer, T., & Sorofman, B. (1988). Minority elderly: Health care and policy issues. In W. Van Horne (Ed.), *Ethnicity and public policy* (Series 7). Madison: University of Wisconsin Press.

Tripp-Reimer, T., & Sorofman, B. (1989). *Illness related self-care behaviors in four ethnic groups: Final report to the National Center for Nursing Research.* Bethesda, MD: National Institute of Nursing Research.

Ulbrich, P. M., & Bradsher, J. E. (1993). Perceived support, help seeking and adaptation to stress among older black and white women living along. *Journal of Aging and Health, 5,* 365–386.

Ulbrich, P. M., & Warheit, G. J. (1989). Social support, stress and psychological distress among older black and white adults. *Journal of Aging and Health, 1*(3),286–305.

U.S. Bureau of the Census. (1993). *Profiles of America's elderly: Racial and ethnic diversity of America's elderly population* (Pub. No. POP/93-1). Washington, DC: Author.

U.S. Department of Health and Human Services. (1990). *Healthy people 2000: National health promotion and disease prevention objectives* (No. PHS 91–50213). Washington, DC: Author.

Wallace, S. P. (1995). Minority elderly access to long-term care. Research Activities & Agency for Health Care Policy and Research 188: 17.

White-Means, S. I., & Thornton, M. C. (1990). Ethnic differences in the production of informal home health care. *Gerontologist, 30,* 758–768.

Willis, D. (1989). *Health policies and black Americans.* New Brunswick, NJ: Transaction Books.

Wolinsky, F. D., Aguirre, B. E., Faan, L. J., Keith, V. M., Arnold, C. L., Niederhauer, J. C., & Dietrich, K. (1989). Ethnic differences in the demand for physician and hospital utilization among older adults in major American cities: Conspicuous evidence of considerable inequalities. *Milbank Quarterly, 67*(3-4), 412–449.

Wolinsky, F. D., Callahan, C. M., Fitzgerald, J. F., & Johnson, R. J. (1992). The risk of nursing home placement and subsequent death among older adults. *Journal of Gerontology: Social Sciences, 47*(4), S173–S182.

Wray, L. A. (1992). Health policy and ethnic diversity in older Americans: Dissonance or harmony? *Western Journal of Medicine, 157,* 357–361.

Wykle, M., & Kaskel, B. (1991). Increasing the longevity of minority older adults through improved health status. In *Minority elders: Longevity, economics, and health* (pp. 24–32). Washington, DC: Gerontological Society of America.

Yeatts, D., Crow, T., & Folts, E. (1992). Service use among low-income minority elderly: Strategies for overcoming barriers. *Gerontologist, 32*(1), 24–32.

Yeo, G. (1991). Ethnogeriatric education: Need and content. *Journal of Cross-Cultural Gerontology, 6*(2), 229–241.

Zayas, L. H., & Ozuah, P. O. (1996). Mercury use in espiritismo: A survey of botanicas. *American Journal of Public Health, 86*(1), 111–112.

CHAPTER 6

Social Support, Social Networks, and the Problem of Loneliness in Elder Care

Bethel Ann Powers

References to "support networks" or "social support networks" abound in the gerontological literature and often seem to be used interchangeably with concepts of "social support" and "social network." The notion of "support network" reflects convergence in the 1980s of two distinct fields of literature. This chapter begins by briefly reviewing origins of the literatures on social support and social networks and the nature of scholarship in each of these fields. The health and well-being of elders in relation to social support and network issues are addressed next. Finally, the problem of loneliness is considered as an example of an experience not wholly captured by social support and social network approaches. Reflections on this topic stem from serendipitous findings from my previously reported research on social networks of elderly institutionalized people (Powers, 1988a, 1988b, 1991, 1992, 1995). The central point is concerned with the limitations of viewing social network and social support research as a substitute for loneliness research and the importance of studying "up front" the phenomenon of loneliness as experienced by elderly persons.

The experience of chronic illness is unique to the individual and not limited to the pathophysiology of disease. While disease may be the problem from the health care provider's perspective, the issue for older adults with various incurable conditions is how to live with and respond to symptoms and disabilities. What illnesses mean to them from the perspective of their everyday lives will influence their opinions about relative health status and sense of well-being. This discussion focuses on the social dimension of chronic illness, which may be experienced as engagement with members of one's personal network or as isolation from others.

RESEARCH ON SOCIAL SUPPORT AND SOCIAL NETWORKS

Studies of Social Support

The literature on social support derives from the field of community mental health, specifically, the seminal work of John Cassel, an epidemiologist, and Gerald Caplan, a social psychiatrist. Cassel (1974) hypothesized about the health-protective role of social contact as a moderator of stress. Caplan (1974) elaborated on Cassel's theoretical formulations of psychosocial processes by classifying types of support systems and outlining activities that community mental health workers could pursue to promote development of supportive attachments. The ideas of Caplan and Cassel about social support and health inspired many empirical studies and action projects and focused future agendas in the areas of stress and coping, life span development and social adaptation, and health services research.

For the past several decades, theorists and researchers across disciplines have argued that social support promotes health and emotional well-being, particularly in the presence of stressful circumstances (Bloom, 1990; Callaghan & Morrissey, 1993; Cohen & Syme, 1985; Gottlieb, 1981; Yarcheski, Scolovino, & Mahon, 1994). Heller, Swindle, and Dusenbury (1986) conceptualized the two key components of social support as (1) esteem-enhancing appraisals and (2) stress-related interpersonal transactions. The esteem-enhancing appraisals component draws on symbolic interactionists' interpretations of how people's self-concept is shaped by their perceptions of their worth, value, likableness, or importance to others. Perceived support depends on individuals' abilities to evaluate personal relationships and suggests mutuality, with or without actual resource exchange. The stress-related interpersonal transactions component draws on the coping literature and theories about the stress-buffering effects of support (Thoits, 1986). Support in this instance depends on resources available to an individual from others that, in addition to being available, can also be mobilized. According to Heller et al., social support influences health and well-being not through its presence but in the way it is perceived. Consequently, it cannot be assessed apart from the meaning of relationships and activities to individuals.

Investigations of social support typically have focused attention on the situational contexts of stressful events, personality variables, or quality and quantity of social contacts. While there is no commonly agreed-upon definition of social support, types of support (e.g., informational, emotional, material) have been identified (Jacobson, 1986; Schwarzer & Leppin, 1991) and researchers have examined perceived benefits of multidimensional aspects of support in a variety of health-related situations (Dunkel-Schetter & Wortman, 1982; Gulick, 1994; King, Reis, Porter, & Norsen, 1993; Lehman, Ellard, & Wortman, 1986; Logsdon, McBride, & Birkimer, 1994; Murata, 1994; Norbeck, Chaftez, Skodel-Wilson, & Weiss, 1991; Stewart, 1989; Yates, 1995).

In contrast to the focus on positive aspects of supportive behaviors, there is rising interest in how negative aspects of social interaction affect perceptions of social support (Coyne & Downey, 1991; Finch, Okun, Barrera, & Zautra, 1989; Krause, 1995; Krause & Jay, 1991; Pagel, Erdly, & Becker, 1987; Rook, 1984, 1990). Work in this area suggests that satisfaction with received support is more likely to occur when negative interactions with network members can be avoided. Reciprocal relationships, in which older adults are giving as well as receiving support, are of particular interest because of the increased exposure to the negative side of social encounters that accompanies benefits from being more actively involved with others. "These mixed findings seem to be more consistent with recently emerging views of the social support process as a tenuous balance between concern and resentment as well as intimacy and conflict" (Krause, 1955, p. 70).

Social Network Studies

Social network theory defines social support as contingent resources flowing through sets of interpersonal ties that connect network members to a focal individual and to each other. Analysis of personal networks thus includes an examination of ways in which network member interactions affect the flow of resources to the focal individual. Description is concerned with patterns of relationships among network members rather than with personal characteristics of individuals. Resources can be measured in terms of (a) *content* (specifically defined resources, e.g., tangible types of assistance, emotional attachment, or companionship), (b) *quantity* (frequency and amount of resources flowing in any direction), (c) *quality* (perceived intensity of the relationship and satisfaction with the content of resource exchange), (d) *multiplexity* (whether the tie provides one or more types of resources), and (e) *directionality* (whether resource exchange tends to be reciprocal or whether resources tend to flow only in one direction). In addition to the previously described interactional characteristics of networks, analysis of network data also involves description of structural characteristics: (a) *size* (total number of active ties), (b) *homogeneity* (similarity of network member attributes), (c) *density* and *interconnectedness* (nature and extent of relationships that members of a focal individual's network have with others in the same network), (d) *clustering* (network segments that not only have high density but also common interaction), and (e) *content dispersion* (ratio of actual to potential number of activity fields from which network members are drawn) (Sokolovsky, 1980).

The literature on social networks derives from social science field investigations of human organization. Barnes (1954), in a report of an anthropological study of Norwegian fishing village groups, was the first to describe social networks as types of informal ties of friendship, kinship, and acquaintanceship that reach across but are not readily subsumed by formal groups or categories. Subsequent urban and family studies in anthropology established the social network concept by calling attention to its importance in organizing social life and by developing ways to measure the structural properties and interactional characteristics of networks (Bott, 1957; Mayer, 1966; Mitchell, 1969; Sanjek, 1978). Urban sociologists, coming to the study of networks from a different methodological perspective, used algebraic algorithms and developed sociometric techniques to depict patterns in personal network structures graphically (Fischer, 1976; Wellman & Leighton, 1979). They also studied ways in which individuals gained resources through the mobilization of network ties (Bernard & Killworth, 1978; Granovetter, 1974; Lee, 1969).

Questions about how the structure and content of personal ties affect the flow of resources to the focal individual encouraged the convergence of social network theory and studies of social support. However, Wellman (1981) took issue with (1) support system studies that invoke the "social network" metaphor to refer to sets of loosely defined supportive relationships while ignoring network analysis approaches, and (2) a preoccupation with "support" networks, particularly when applied to personal networks in their entirety. He argued that "focus on a simple support/nonsupport dichotomy de-emphasizes the multifaceted, often contradictory nature of social ties" (p. 173). To this end, he pointed out that not all network relationships are necessarily supportive; that, likely, only a third of one's network is apt to be available for help in an emergency and less will be available on a day-to-day basis; and that mobilization of support is variously affected by such network characteristics as density and the relative strength of interpersonal ties.

SOCIAL SUPPORT AND HEALTH STATUS OF ELDERS

Research consistently suggests that social support is important and figures positively in the well-being of elderly persons, who are at increased risk for illness and disruption of natural support systems caused by such stressful events as retirement, relocation, and death of spouses and contemporaries (Bear, 1990a, 1990b; Eckert, 1983; Friedman, 1993; Glicksman, Lazarus, Wilson, & Leeder, 1995; Kelman, Thomas, & Tanaka, 1994; McIntosh, Kaplan, Kubena, & Landmann, 1993; Mor-Barak, Scharlach, Birba, & Sokolovsky, 1992; Peterson & Quadagno, 1985; Pilisuk & Minkler, 1980; Pohl & Fuller, 1980; Rubinstein, 1985; Seeman & Berkman, 1988; Van Willigen, 1989). Minkler (1985) noted an absence of evidence to support the idea that the relationship among social networks, social support, and health status is different for elders than for other age groups. However, elders are disproportionately affected by chronic illness, which does increase demands on support systems over time. Filinson (1985) suggested that chronic illness care tends to be "removed from the public arena and privatized, as the patient and his or her social support network construct their own idiosyncratic modes of dealing with the disease" (p. 326). As the curative role of medicine recedes, personal care services to support independent functioning gain in importance, with long-term assistance falling by default on familial and informal support systems. Elders with limited personal and financial resources are particularly vulnerable.

Frail Elders Living Alone

Rubinstein and his colleagues (Rubinstein, 1986; Rubinstein, Kilbride, & Nagy, 1992) have conducted extensive field research on frail elders living alone in a large American city and surrounding suburbs. A detailed investigation of 47 older men (Rubinstein, 1986) revealed individual variation in personal routines, levels of activity, and patterns of social contact. Roughly half ("nonisolates") attended a senior center or were residents in senior-only housing units, while the other half ("isolates") were not so connected. Anthropological methods of participant observation and in-depth interviewing were used to elicit information. The meaning of living alone that emerged from the stories of these men was discussed in relation to contrasting and noncontrasting themes. Contrasting themes represented issue-oriented possibilities that were understood and responded to by participants in individualistic ways. The issues concerned sense of independence versus feelings of being "tied down"; control or lack of control over life; social equity or inequity; activity or inactivity; familial connectedness or family apartness; and relative value of present versus past in current daily life. Noncontrasting themes represented common areas of individual meaning attached to living alone (family, spouse, home, present-day evaluation of the past, and daily scheduling of activities). Rubinstein found that no life transition was as important to men who had been married as was widowhood in late life. Additionally, in the case of bachelors, a particular type of late life devastation was described that was distinctive from widowhood and was characterized by much unhappiness, stress, conflict, and ambiguity. The loneliness and disconnectedness experienced by many of the men in the study was thought to be tied directly to an inability to reorganize their lives successfully after the loss of significant network ties (spouse, parent, close friend, or family member).

Another field study of 52 male and female frail and functionally impaired elders living alone (Rubinstein et al., 1992) examined environmental factors that contribute to independence and, hence, successful aging. The majority of participants had a number of difficult health situations, with large percentages suffering from heart problems, hypertension, circulatory disease, and arthritis. Many also complained about difficulty with sleeping, nervousness, and tension. Through case presentation, participants accounted for choices they had had within the physical and social environments of home and neighborhood. Their experiences with making choices linked to independence and successful aging were described collectively as "a balancing act" resting on their abilities to be accepting of much that was not well in their lives. Resourcefulness that compensates for diminished networks and sources of informal support comes at a price. The researchers stated: "We are concerned here with what we call the *miniaturization of satisfaction.* By this we mean, that for our impaired informants at least, the realm of those factors that contribute to a sense of well-being or that mitigate difficulties is small, circumspect, and at hand. Decisions about satisfaction are not based in the realm of big choices or possibilities but in the realm of small events" (Rubenstein et al., p. 143). An underlying critical concern of the research is "with the nature of American culture and the burdens it places on the individual, even the individual whose situation is grossly compromised, to provide for personal agency unassisted. And personal agency is increasingly economic and materialistic and the formal solutions increasingly cosmetic" (p. 155). [The concept of "personal agency" has to do with self-responsibility; capacity or power to make choices, and to be in control of one's life; ability to operate independently/independent living.]

Taken as a whole, these reports of frail elders living alone present portraits that "smooth the desperation and conflict in which many of [the] informants lived" without masking observed "deep structural inequalities based on wealth, access to resources, and the political economy of choice" (Rubinstein et al., 1992, p. 153). They illustrate graphically the imposing realities of cultural, social, and political environments that make it difficult for many elders to obtain the resources that will enable them to continue living in their own communities.

Elderly Loners and the Homeless

Sokolovsky and Cohen's social network studies (1981, 1983) have focused on support systems of inner-city single room occupancy (SRO) aged and elderly homeless men (Sokolovsky & Cohen, 1981, 1983; Cohen & Sokolovsky, 1989). Personal ties of 96 men and women living in 11 SRO hotels were surveyed (Sokolovsky & Cohen, 1981, 1983) using a network profile interview guide designed to elicit objective and subjective measures of social interaction (Sokolovsky, 1980). The hotel environment as described was drab, depressing, and dangerous. Participants were from hotel populations that included high percentages of the mentally disturbed and the physically deteriorated with multiple chronic illnesses and a high rate of alcoholism.

It was found that many of these self-proclaimed loners had widely dispersed and larger than expected networks, but there was a reluctance to acknowledge the significance of relationships and a tendency to activate ties selectively to meet needs (e.g., visiting, food preparation/borrowing, money loans, shopping, illness care), while avoiding intimacy and limiting involvement with societal institutions. Thus some individuals maintained support systems that afforded a minimum of physical and social contact, but with so few sources of help on which to depend that a sudden loss or crisis would leave them extremely vulnerable.

"From a certain perspective which measures cultural meaning by group-oriented activity the SRO elderly would indeed be isolated" (Sokolovsky & Cohen, 1983, p. 201). The study revealed, however, that despite relatively low levels of social interaction, SRO aged were able to create and maintain systems of personal support. Remaining was the issue of vulnerability, given the absence in so many networks of instrumentally and emotionally important ties, very low frequency of contact with kin, and avoidance of formal support services. This, researchers claimed, made it difficult to evaluate whether or not or to what extent the SRO elderly were truly isolated. That they had few viable options was clear, though:

> Most aged realize that if they are not able to maintain themselves in the SRO, a nursing home or perhaps skid row are the only alternatives, a thought which strikes terror in their hearts. (Sokolovsky & Cohen, 1983, p. 195)

In the second study (Cohen & Sokolovsky, 1989), 177 of the 281 homeless old men who were interviewed lived in flophouses, 86 lived on the street, and the remaining 18 lived in apartments. In addition to the network profile, an instrument that has been used cross-nationally to assess physical health, psychiatric symptoms, and the social and economic needs of geriatric populations was employed. All of the men were in poor physical health with a high rate of ambulatory and hearing difficulties, respiratory and somatic symptoms, edema, hypertension, and gastrointestinal complaints. Some (23%) demonstrated overt psychotic behavior or acknowledged past psychiatric hospitalization, but only 3% reported that they were taking medication for mental or emotional problems. Depression and physical symptoms frequently occurred together and were most associated with an inability to meet daily needs. Except in the cases of a few men who seemed to be true isolates, social support for about two-thirds of the men included passing time or exchanging conversation, food, and drink in small social groups of about three or four individuals, as well as involvement with formal agencies (e.g., food programs, missions, shelters, and donated services) for about two-thirds of the men. Although more accepting of services and more sociable overall than the SRO elderly, these homeless elderly were trapped in a downward spiral of diminishing resources. The researchers warned that they represent the future for young homeless people if appropriate intervention is not forthcoming:

> We have described the effects of living in the squalor of skid row. The effects on the body and soul further serve to entrench these men there. Possibilities for employment become even more limited in our society as these men become physically frailer and older. Most of these men are considered "old" by 50. Their lives mirror those of persons in third world countries who prematurely age as they are caught in the inescapable cycle of poverty. (Cohen & Sokolovsky, 1989, p. 218)

The previous studies demonstrate the resourcefulness of the SRO and homeless elderly in terms of minimally meeting needs for sustenance and casual human contact through creation and maintenance of small utilitarian networks. However, individuals' informal networks left little to fall back upon in time of crisis. Organized, coordinated formal support available to poor urban elderly at the most basic level remains woefully insufficient.

Institutionalized Elders

Sokolovsky's network profile approach (1980) also was used in Powers's study of elderly institutionalized people (Powers, 1988a, 1988b, 1991, 1992, 1995). Data were gathered on all direct contacts that the 69 male and female participants had with people in and outside of the institution. The profile involved four sectors of interaction: resident-resident, resident-staff, resident-kin, and resident-outside friend or acquaintance. Four types of networks were identified, differing in terms of size, clustering of ties, interconnectedness, and interactional characteristics.

1. *Institution-centered networks* were small with proportionally fewer outside as opposed to intrainstitutional contacts. Ties were often simple and of low intensity. Self-proclaimed "loners" developed their own routines that brought them into contact with individuals within the institution who could meet needs for passing time or supplying tangible goods and services with a minimal amount of emotional involvement. High value was placed on self-reliance, accompanied by resistance to bureaucratic control. In contrast, those in the group who were isolated due to loss of a highly support-

ive outside person were more apt to turn to staff as a source of dependent support and emotional attachment.

2. *Small cluster networks* were variants of institution-centered networks that contained small cliques of residents who regularly spent time together and shared confidences with one another.

3. In *kin-centered networks,* residents had an average of four relatives who visited and communicated with them on a weekly or monthly basis. Emotional ties to families made it difficult for some residents to accept institutional relationships or activities.

4. Last, *balanced networks* were the largest in size and demonstrated the greatest interconnectedness. A wide range of contacts across the different sectors of resident, staff, kin, and outside friend or acquaintance facilitated the flow of communication and support.

This research demonstrated the diversity of institutionalized elderly. Some residents' network interactions reflected a continuation of patterns from their earlier lives. Others had experienced network changes from previous periods either through loss or through new opportunities for relationship formation. (For example, one study participant in a small cluster network, who had remained at home all her life, in the end caring for her aged parents, remarked, "I never had a social life before I came here.") In different studies involving network typologies, there is evidence to suggest that some network types may develop out of other types in response to changes across individuals' life spans, such as geographic relocation or death of important network members (Wenger, 1989). In this research, the kin-centered network may be a transitional type out of which institution-centered, small cluster, or balanced networks evolve if residents become increasingly disengaged from kin ties as a result of diminished contact over time.

Attention so often is called to the institutionalized elders' lack of support systems and social network ties. Appreciating the dynamic nature of networks and the active ways in which residents shape and maintain network relationships brings into sharper focus the dimension of informal support activities that operates outside of formal systems. Sensitivity to what residents need and seek in terms of social support also involves appreciation of the diversity in network types and openness to what individuals' network arrangements may reveal about lifestyle patterns and preferences that are important to them. Knowledge of personal networks permits avoidance of interference where support is strong and concentration of assistanc(where lack of support is observed.

ISSUES IN THE STUDY OF SOCIAL SUPPORT IN LATER LIFE

Conceptual Issues

Concerns about direction and progress in the study of social support focus both on conceptual and methodological issues. Conceptually, there is the business of separating the components of social support (Lieberman, 1986). To plan effective interventions, it may be important to be able to match types of support that have been found to be useful with the particular needs associated with different stressful circumstances. Various typologies of supportive behaviors have been proposed, and work continues on specifying which supportive acts cause direct or buffering effects on health. Questions regarding the roles of age, sex, culture, and personality in the relationship between social support and health also continue to be pursued. For example, Jacobson (1987) discussed the influence of cultural context in relation to support networks of 20 noninstitutionalized elderly men and women. Additionally, while there is evidence of a strong association between social support and mental health, linkages between social support and physical health (e.g., influence on the immune system or on other biological processes that trigger physiological responses to disease) continue to be a challenging area to assess (McIntosh et al., 1993).

Understanding the relationship between satisfaction with social support and well-being raises additional conceptual issues. Research has suggested that subjective perceptions of social network relationships and personal satisfaction with received support are more strongly related to psychological well-being than objective measures of the social support process, such as number of personal ties and frequency of interaction with others (Krause, 1989; Krause, Liang, & Yatomi, 1989). Krause's (1995) conceptual model of satisfaction with support in later life contrasts two factors said to influence perceived support. The first factor is the actual amount of assistance and support received. Receiving assistance may produce satisfaction in the form of feedback to individuals that they are valued and that their networks are functioning adequately. The second factor is based on the works of Rook (1984, 1990) and others (e.g., Krause & Jay, 1991; Pagel et al., 1987), which examine the impact of negative interactions on satisfaction with support. A test of the model using data from a nationwide survey of older adults suggested that negative interaction is more strongly related to satisfaction with support than measures of received support and that the impact of both of these factors depends, in turn, upon the amount of reciprocal exchange between elders and members of their networks (Krause, 1995).

> The notion that satisfaction with support is determined by negative interaction has profound implications for the way that we think about the social support process. As Coyne and Downey (1991) point out, this perspective tends to turn the concept of social support on its head. Instead of arising from the helpful behaviors, the benefits of associating with others may be attributed to the ability of social network members to stave off or avert negative interaction. This alternative view suggests that those who develop interventions to bolster natural support systems may need to reconceptualize the basic thrust of their programs. Rather than attempting to encourage supportive behaviors, these practitioners may want to focus on eradicating negative or upsetting interaction. (Krause, p. 59)

In service of a more complete or comprehensive conceptualization of social support processes in later life, more needs to be learned about relationships among received support, negative interaction, reciprocity, and satisfaction with social support.

Methodological Issues

Methodologically, absence of common operational definitions of social support and the variety of measurement approaches used make across-study comparisons difficult. Since much reported research has been correlational in design, the need to generate causal explanations of the relationship of social support to health through greater use of experimental approaches has been emphasized (Bloom, 1990; Callaghan & Morrissey, 1993). To balance heavy reliance on cross-sectional self-report questionnaire data, there have been recommendations for the increased use of multidimensional, longitudinal study approaches that attempt to capture more fully the complex, changing, and fluid nature of support that occurs over time (Bloom, 1990; Lieberman, 1986). Social network mapping and qualitative approaches involving participant observation and in-depth interviewing continue to be useful in describing network structure, detailing the dynamics of interaction within networks, and eliciting individuals' perceptions of supportive and nonsupportive aspects of relationships.

Over the years, progress in the study of social support has been linked with needs to achieve consensus in defining and measuring the concept and to account theoretically for its impact on health. Reviewers of this literature encourage further exploration in the previously described directions while exercising caution over more than tentative assertions about the role and importance of support (Bloom, 1990; Callaghan & Morrissey, 1993).

> To study the major unanswered research questions in the relation of social support to health requires further explication of the concept of social support itself and consistent assessment of current measurement tools. Thus, the explanation as to how support comes to effect health is another potentially fruitful line of inquiry . . . [that] should be a high priority for a research agenda for the nineties. (Bloom, p. 636)

THE PROBLEM OF LONELINESS

The problem of loneliness in old age has been linked with social isolation or subsumed under quality of life issues pertaining to social engagement (Berg, Mellstrom, Persson, & Svanborg, 1981; Blau, 1961; Clark, 1971; Creecy, Berg, & Wright, 1985; Lowenthal, 1964; Mor et al., 1995; Rubinstein, 1985, 1986; Rubinstein et al., 1992; Stephans & Bernstein, 1984; Stephens, 1976; Townsend, 1968; Turnstall, 1967). Objective factors considered in attempts to explain the loneliness of social isolation have included demographic and ecological variables that affect social relationships, such as network density, network changes in response to life course events, geographical distance from family and close friends, or types of living arrangements. From this perspective, the emphasis is on the extent and nature of personal ties and on the processes involved in mobilizing and directing support to individuals through formal and personal network systems. However, the broader phenomenon of loneliness has not been well studied.

Jones (1989) identified "the tendency to view loneliness as a substitute measure of the quality and quantity of an individual's relationships" as a major problem in loneliness research and asserted that the "study of loneliness is the study of an internal syndrome or state and not the study of relationships" (pp. 28–29). Social isolation that results from absence of community, or disengagement from a social network, is qualitatively different from the emotional isolation that results from absence of attachment figures (Weiss, 1973). The anxiety of social isolation is provoked by a sense of vulnerability: "It isn't missing the fun that leads to the loneliness of social isolation; it's being on your own, without allies, in a dangerous world" (Weiss, 1989, p. 13). The distress of emotional isolation is triggered by loss of or changes in relationships with individuals perceived as sources of emotional security (Weiss, 1973, 1989).

Participants in Powers's study of elderly institutionalized people's social networks (1988a, 1988b, 1991, 1992, 1995) spoke of loneliness as a subjective feeling or emotion. While elicitation of network data was the focus of the research, a conversational interviewing style facilitated collection of other kinds of information, including responses to the question "Are you ever lonely?" The responses to this question have not been reported previously.

Out of 69 participants, 37 (54%) said they were never lonely and 32 (46%) claimed to be lonely sometimes. When residents elaborated on the experience of loneliness, some complained about boredom or not enough socializing (social isolation). But the majority of descriptions of what loneliness was like for individuals involved emotional isolation—grieving past separations and losses, as illustrated by the following examples drawn from interview transcripts and fieldnotes:

> Example (institution-centered network): I used to have good friends, but I haven't seen these so-called friends in 4 to 6 months. That schooled me pretty good. When I get back [to the low-income hotel], I won't remember them neither. You know, if you don't give the kid no candy, he won't be looking. It's kinda lonesome, but you don't want to let nothing bother you too much.

This man bitterly mourned the loss of companions to whom he longed to return. He also expressed the idea that offering friendship ("candy") creates expectations that lead to disappointment if the sweetness is withheld.

> Example (small cluster network): I get lonesome [for them]. I miss my old friends terribly.

This participant was a member of a close group of residents who "chummed around together." While needs for socialization reportedly were satisfied, missing old friends "terribly" was part of a lingering sadness associated with memories of preinstitutional life.

> Example (kin-centered network): I got used to it [being lonesome and missing family]; [and now] I don't care anymore.

The lonesomeness of this participant was experienced as despair over physical separation from family members and resistance to the idea that returning home might be an unrealistic expectation.

> Example (balanced network): I don't require what so many others require. They're lonesome if nobody's with 'em. As for me, I like to be by myself, but my wife—that's the one I miss.

The pain of bereavement was recent for this participant. His wife had been a resident in the institution as well, and together they had a wide variety of social ties. However, she primarily maintained their social network, while his attention and activities focused more on her.

While patterns of social interaction differed by network type, with balanced networks exhibiting the least degree of social isolation and institution-centered networks containing more social isolates, no particular network configuration served to counteract the experience of emotional isolation. Weiss (1973) has commented on the greater ease of relieving the loneliness of social isolation by enhancing social networks in contrast to alleviating the loneliness of emotional isolation, where new relationships would need to approximate more closely the intensity of those that had been lost.

And what of those residents who claimed never to be lonely? There could be a variety of explanations. They might have been lonely but unwilling to admit it. They might have been unaware of being lonely if the loneliness was masked by other responses such as depression, anxiety, or anger (Perlman & Joshi, 1989), or they might in fact not have been lonely. Loneliness is not the same as aloneness. Early theorists have stressed the importance of distinguishing loneliness from solitude. Peplau (1955) emphasized that persons who choose to be alone for specific purposes may not experience loneliness. Consequently, a person could have few social contacts and yet seldom feel lonely; other persons could have many personal ties and be very active socially while simultaneously experiencing feelings of loneliness.

Whether or not elderly people suffer more from loneliness than other age groups is not clear (Rubinstein, 1986). A better understanding of the phenomenon and how it affects individuals across the life course is needed. However, one difficulty in understanding the experience of loneliness is lack of consensus on the definition and measurement of the concept. Because loneliness is an internal, subjective state, its essence is not likely to be captured through an explanation of social relationships. Existing measurements, such as the UCLA Loneliness Scale (Russell, 1982), have been useful but also criticized for incompletely approximating the experience without accounting for what it means to different persons in different circumstances. It has been suggested that phenomenological methods would be especially suited to extend understanding of "the various types of loneliness; the relation of loneliness to other affective states, like depression, anxiety, and self-esteem; the nature of attachment relationships, feeling vulnerable, and feeling lonely" (Stokes, 1989, p. 61). Johnson and Mullins (1987) also emphasized the value of a phenomenological (experiential) approach in distinguishing between aloneness and loneliness and in sorting out different types of subjective loneliness. This approach does not discount the idea of a relationship between social isolation and the experience of loneliness or the usefulness of social support and social network approaches to evaluate this dimension, but such evaluations will be limited and may fail to capture and faithfully convey the experiential aspects of the loneliness phenomenon. An understanding of the whole experience is essential for accurate assessment of people's varying needs and for the creation of meaningful interventions that will enhance elderly individuals' abilities to cope with loneliness.

While interest in studying social support has been sustained over a number of years, loneliness research has seemed to wax and wane. In reflecting on my own social network data and after surveying some of the loneliness literature, I am more convinced than ever of the need to study loneliness "up front," building on existing loneliness theory, and using a variety of approaches to understand better the interplay between the objective and subjective components of this multidimensional concept.

CONCLUSION

Social support is important to the health and well-being of elderly people, who are at increased risk for illness and disruption of natural support systems. Some examples of research with particularly vulnerable populations—frail elders living alone, elderly loners and homeless, and institutionalized elderly—have been presented.

For decades, the study of social support has engaged the attention of a variety of health and social science professionals such as anthropologists, epidemiologists, gerontologists, nurses, physicians, public health personnel, psychologists, and sociologists. Additionally, approaches from the field of social network research have enhanced understanding of social support by providing a means to describe and measure interaction and resource exchange within the web of personal relationships that individuals maintain over time. Although there is consensus on the multidimensional nature of social support and its importance in promoting health and well-being, arriving at a unified definition of the concept, common measurement approaches, and explanations of its role in promoting mental and physical health remains a challenge. There has been a call for more emphasis on experimental and multidimensional longitudinal studies. Continued research on negative interaction in later life is particularly important, since elders may have lessened ability to remove themselves from problematic encounters (Krause, 1995, p. 71). The kinds of relationships most prone to negative interactions (e.g., family relationships) need to be more thoroughly researched. Conceptualization of the social support process also requires a balancing of objective facts and subjective perceptions about the amount, availability, and adequacy of support that imply a need to employ a variety of study approaches, both quantitative and qualitative.

Typologies of support have been proposed, and work continues on specifying which supportive acts have direct and/or buffering effects on health. At the same time, the influence of negative interaction on satisfaction with social support has begun to be more appreciated. Clearly, not all interaction within social networks is positive and assistive. Some relationships may be a burden; some interactions may be upsetting even in the presence of resource exchange. The view that negative interaction may have more effect on satisfaction with support than the actual amount of assistance received suggests a redirection of thinking about interventions to strengthen natural support systems, that is, efforts might need to expand from a narrow focus on promotion of supportive behaviors to include attempts at reducing upsetting interactions.

Social isolation, particularly interpersonal isolation from family, friends, and workplace, has been studied in connection with emphases on needs for increased support and reinforcement of networks. Prevention of social isolation has been viewed as a way to address the problem of loneliness. It has been argued here, however, that loneliness is no more a unidimensional concept than is the concept of social support. Consequently, although the loneliness of social isolation may be one component of the loneliness experience, it cannot be used to explain the whole or different manifestations of this phenomenon. In addition, objective measures of the quality and quantity of individuals' relationships should not be viewed as substitute measures of loneliness, which has been described as an internal subjective state. Here the limitations of social support and social network research may be noted, and a return to loneliness theory and research to explore more fully the problem of loneliness for elders is urged. Much remains that is not understood about the experience of loneliness. There are recent examples of loneliness research, such as Dugan and Kivett's (1994) study of "the importance of emotional and social isolation to loneliness among very old rural adults." However, theory building seems to have peaked in the past decade (Hojat & Crandall, 1989). Advancement of this field should be encouraged.

Overall, knowledge of social support is growing despite differences in conceptualization, definition of terms, measurement methods, populations studied, and disciplinary commitments. This diversity itself may be thought of as an enrichment in that the consistencies and patterns that emerge over time may prove more meaningful than conclusions resulting from a narrower, more unified, approach (Cohen & Syme, 1985, p. xvii). There needs to be appreciation for both the strengths and limitations of this field in terms of what may be learned about human bonds and interaction and how those understandings may be applied to benefit elders and other populations, particularly in the promotion of health and wellness.

REFERENCES

Barnes, J. A. (1954). Class and committees in a Norwegian island parish. *Human Relations, 7,* 39–58.

Bear, M. (1990a). Social networks and health: Impact on returning home after entry into residential care homes. *Gerontologist, 30,* 30–34.

Bear, M. (1990b). Social network characteristics and the duration of primary relationships after entry into long-term care. *Journal of Gerontology, 45,* S156–S162.

Berg, S., Mellstrom, D., Persson, G., & Svanborg, A. (1981). Loneliness in the Swedish aged. *Journal of Gerontology, 36,* 342–349.

Bernard, H. R., & Killworth, P. A. (1978). A review of the small world literature. *Connections, 2,* 15–24.

Blau, Z. (1961). Structural constraints of friendship in old age. *American Sociological Review, 26,* 429–439.

Bloom, J. R. (1990). The relationship of social support and health. *Social Science & Medicine, 30,* 635–637.

Bott, E. (1957). *Family and social network.* London: Tavistock.

Callaghan, P., & Morrissey, J. (1993). Social support and health: A review. *Journal of Advanced Nursing, 18,* 203–210.

Caplan, G. (1974). *Support systems and community mental health.* New York: Basic Books.

Cassel, J. (1974). Psychosocial processes and "stress": Theoretical formulations. *International Journal of Health Services, 4,* 471–482.

Clark, M. (1971). Patterns of aging among elders poor of the inner city. *Gerontologist, 11,* 58–66.

Cohen, C., & Sokolovsky, J. (1989). *Old men of the Bowery: Strategies for survival among the homeless.* New York: Guilford Press.

Cohen, S., & Syme, S. L. (Eds.). (1985). *Social support and health.* Orlando, FL: Academic Press.

Coyne, J. C., & Downey, G. (1991). Social factors and psychopathology: Stress, social support, and coping processes. *Annual Review of Psychology, 42,* 401–425.

Creecy, R. F., Berg, W. E., & Wright, R. (1985). Loneliness among elders: A causal approach. *Journal of Gerontology, 40,* 487–493.

Dugan, M. A., & Kivett, V. R. (1994). The importance of emotional and social isolation to loneliness among very old rural adults. *Gerontologist, 34,* 340–346.

Dunkel-Schetter, C., & Wortman, C. (1982). The interpersonal dynamics of cancer: Problems in social relationships and their impact on the patient. In H. S. Friedman & M. R. DiMatteo (Eds.), *Interpersonal issues in health care* (pp. 69–100). San Diego, CA: Academic Press.

Eckert, J. K. (1983). Dislocation and relocation of the urban elderly: Social networks as mediators of relocation stress. *Human Organization, 42,* 39–56.

Filinson, R. (1985). Chronic illness and care provision: A study of Alzheimer's disease. In W. A. Peterson & J. Quadagno (Eds.), *Social bonds in later life: Aging and interdependence* (pp. 325–347). Beverly Hills, CA: Sage.

Finch, J. F., Okun, M. A., Barrera, M., & Zautra, A. (1989). Positive and negative social ties among older adults. *American Journal of Community Psychology, 17,* 585–605.

Fischer, C. S. (1976). *The urban experience.* New York: Harcourt Brace Jovanovitch.

Friedman, M. M. (1993). Social support sources and psychological well-being in older women with heart disease. *Research in Nursing & Health, 16,* 405–413.

Glicksman, M. D., Lazarus, R., Wilson, A., & Leeder, S. R. (1995). Social support, marital status and living arrangement correlates of cardiovascular disease risk factors in elders. *Social Science & Medicine, 40,* 811–814.

Gottlieb, B. H. (Ed.). (1981). *Social networks and social support.* Beverly Hills, CA: Sage.

Gulick, E. E. (1994). Social support among persons with multiple sclerosis. *Research in Nursing & Health, 17,* 195–206.

Granovetter, M. (1974). *Getting a job.* Cambridge, MA: Harvard University Press.

Heller, K., Swindle, R. W., & Dusenbury, L. (1986). Component social support processes: Comments and integration. *Journal of Consulting and Clinical Psychology, 54,* 466–470.

Hojat, M., & Crandall, R. (Eds.). (1989). *Loneliness: Theory, research, and applications.* Newbury Park, CA: Sage.

Jacobson, D. (1986). Types and timing of social support. *Journal of Health and Social Behavior, 27,* 250–264.

Jacobson, D. (1987). The cultural context of social support and support networks. *Medical Anthropology Quarterly, 1,* 42–67.

Johnson, D. P., & Mullins, L. C. (1987). Growing old and lonely in different societies: Toward a comparative perspective. *Journal of Cross-Cultural Gerontology, 2,* 257–275.

Jones, W. H. (1989). Research and theory on loneliness: A response to Weiss's reflections. In M. Hojat & R. Crandall (Eds.), *Loneliness: Theory, research, and applications* (pp. 27–30). Newbury Park, CA: Sage.

Kelman, H. R., Thomas, C., & Tanaka, J. S. (1994). Longitudinal patterns of formal and informal social support in an urban elderly population. *Social Science & Medicine, 38,* 905–914.

King, K. B., Reis, H. T., Porter, L. A., & Norsen, L. H. (1993). Social support and long-term recovery from coronary artery surgery: Effects on patients and spouses. *Health Psychology, 12,* 56–63.

Krause, N. (1989). Issues of measurement and analysis in studies of social support, aging, and health. In K. S. Markides & C. L. Cooper (Eds.), *Aging, stress, social support, and health* (pp. 43–66). London: John Wiley.

Krause, N. (1995). Negative interaction and satisfaction with social support among older adults. *Journal of Gerontology: Psychological Sciences, 50B,* P59–P73.

Krause, N., & Jay, G. (1991). Stress, social support, and negative interaction in later life. *Research on Aging, 13,* 333–363.

Krause, N., Liang, J., & Yatomi, N. (1989). Satisfaction with social support and depressive symptoms. *Psychology and Aging, 4,* 88–97.

Lee (Howell), N. (1969). *The search for an abortionist.* Chicago: University of Chicago Press.

Lehman, D. R., Ellard, J. H., & Wortman, C. B. (1986). Social support for the bereaved: Recipients' and providers' perspectives on what is helpful. *Journal of Consulting and Clinical Psychology, 54,* 438–446.

Lieberman, M. A. (1986). Social supports—The consequences of psychologizing: A commentary. *Journal of Consulting and Clinical Psychology, 54,* 461–465.

Logsdon, M. C., McBride, A. B., & Birkimer, J. C. (1994). Social support and postpartum depression. *Research in Nursing & Health, 17,* 449–457.

Lowenthal, M. (1964). Social isolation and mental illness in old age. *American Sociological Review, 29,* 54–70.

Mayer, A. C. (1966). The significance of quasi-groups in the study of complex societies. In M. Banton (Ed.), *The social anthropology of complex societies* (pp. 97–122). London: Tavistock.

McIntosh, W. A., Kaplan, H. B., Kubena, K. S., & Landmann, W. A. (1993). Life events, social support, and immune response in elderly individuals. *International Journal of Aging and Human Development, 37,* 23–36.

Minkler, M. (1985). Social support and health of elders. In S. Cohen & S. L. Syme (Eds.), *Social support and health* (pp. 199–216). Orlando, FL: Academic Press.

Mitchell, J. C. (Ed.). (1969). *Social networks in urban situations.* Manchester, England: Manchester University Press.

Mor, V., Branco, K., Fleishman, J., Hawes, C., Phillips, C., Morris, J., & Fries, B. (1995). The structure of social engagement among nursing home residents. *Journal of Gerontology: Psychological Sciences, 50B,* P1–P8.

Mor-Barak, M. E., Scharlach, A. E., Birba, L., & Sokolovsky, J. (1992). Employment, social networks and health in the retirement years. *International Journal of Aging and Human Development, 35,* 145–159.

Murata, J. (1994). Family, stress, social support, violence, and son's behavior. *Western Journal of Nursing Research, 16,* 154–168.

Norbeck, J. S., Chaftez, L., Skodel-Wilson, H., & Weiss, S. J. (1991). Social support needs of family caregivers of psychiatric patients from three age groups. *Nursing Research, 40,* 208–213.

Pagel, M. D., Erdly, W. W., & Becker, J. (1987). Social networks: We get by with (in spite of) a little help from our friends. *Journal of Personality and Social Psychology, 53,* 793–804.

Peplau, H. E. (1955). Loneliness. *American Journal of Nursing, 55,* 1476–1481.

Perlman, D., & Joshi, P. (1989). The revelation of loneliness. In M. Hojat & R. Crandall (Eds.), *Loneliness: Theory, research, and applications* (pp. 63–76). Newbury Park, CA: Sage.

Peterson, W. A., & Quadagno, J. (Eds.). (1985). *Social bonds in later life: Aging and interdependence.* Beverly Hills, CA: Sage.

Pilisuk, M., & Minkler, M. (1980). Supportive networks: Life ties for elders. *Journal of Social Issues, 36,* 95–116.

Pohl, J., & Fuller, S. (1980). Perceived choice, social interaction and dimensions of morale of residents in a home for the aged. *Research in Nursing & Health, 3,* 147–157.

Powers, B. A. (1988a). Self-perceived health of elderly institutionalized people. *Journal of Cross-Cultural Gerontology, 3,* 299–321.

Powers, B. A. (1988b). Social networks, social support, and elderly institutionalized people. *Advances in Nursing Science, 10*(2), 40–58.

Powers, B. A. (1991). The meaning of nursing home friendships. *Advances in Nursing Science, 14*(2), 42–58.

Powers, B. A. (1992). The roles staff play in the social networks of elderly people. *Social Science & Medicine, 34,* 1335–1343.

Powers, B. A. (1995). From the inside out: The world of the institutionalized elderly. In J. N. Henderson & M. D. Vesperi (Eds.), *The culture of long term care: Nursing home ethnography* (pp. 179–196). Westport, CT: Bergin & Garvey.

Rook, K. S. (1984). The negative side of social interaction: Impact on psychological well-being. *Journal of Personality and Social Psychology, 46,* 1097–1108.

Rook, K. S. (1990). Stressful aspects of older adults' social relationships: Current theory and research. In M. A. P. Stephens, J. H. Crowther, S. E. Hobfoll, & D. L. Tennenbaum (Eds.), *Stress and coping in later life families* (pp. 173–192). New York: Hemisphere.

Rubinstein, R. L. (1985). The elderly who live alone and their social supports. In M. P. Lawton & G. L. Maddox (Eds.), *Annual review of gerontology and geriatrics* (pp. 165–193). New York: Springer.

Rubinstein, R. L. (1986). *Singular paths: Old men living alone.* New York: Columbia University Press.

Rubinstein, R. L., Kilbride, J. C., & Nagy, S. (1992). *Elders living alone: Frailty and the perception of choice.* New York: Aldine De Gruyter.

Russell, D. (1982). The measure of loneliness. In L. A. Peplau & D. Perlman (Eds.), *Loneliness: A sourcebook of current theory, research and therapy* (pp. 81–104). New York: John Wiley.

Sanjek, R. A. (1978). A network method and its use in urban ethnography. *Human Organization, 37,* 257–269.

Schwarzer, R., & Leppin, A. (1991). Social support and health: A theoretical and empirical overview. *Journal of Social and Personal Relationships, 8,* 99–127.

Seeman, T. E., & Berkman, L. F. (1988). Structural characteristics of social networks and their relationship with social support in elders: Who provides support? *Social Science & Medicine, 26,* 737–749.

Sokolovsky, J. (1980). Interactional dimensions of the aged: Social network mapping. In C. Fry & J. Keith (Eds.), *New methods for old age research* (pp. 75–100). Chicago: Center for Urban Policy.

Sokolovsky, J., & Cohen, C. (1981). Being old in the inner city: Support systems of the SRO aged. In C. L. Fry (Ed.), *Dimensions: Aging, culture, and health* (pp. 163–184). New York: Praeger.

Sokolovsky, J., & Cohen, C. (1983). Networks as adaptation: The cultural meaning of being a "loner" among the inner-city elderly. In J. Sokolovsky (Ed.), *Growing old in different societies: Cross-cultural perspectives* (pp. 189–201). Belmont, CA: Wadsworth.

Stephans, M. A. P., & Bernstein, M. (1984). Social support and well-being among residents of planned housing. *Gerontologist, 24,* 144–148.

Stephens, J. (1976). *Loners, losers, and lovers: A sociological study of the aged tenants of a slum hotel.* Seattle: University of Washington Press.

Stewart, M. J. (1989). Social support instruments created by nurse investigators. *Nursing Research, 38,* 268–275.

Stokes, J. P. (1989). On the usefulness of phenomenological methods. In M. Hojat & R. Crandall (Eds.), *Loneliness: Theory, research, and applications* (pp. 57–62). Newbury Park, CA: Sage.

Thoits, P. A. (1986). Social support as coping assistance. *Journal of Consulting and Clinical Psychology, 54,* 416–423.

Townsend, P. (1968). Isolation, desolation and loneliness. In E. Shanas, P. Townsend, D. Wedderburn, H. Friis, P. Milhoy, & J. Stehouwer (Eds.), *Old people in three industrial societies* (pp. 258–287). New York: Atherton Press.

Turnstall, J. (1967). *Old and alone.* New York: Humanities Press.

Van Willigen, J. (1989). *Gettin' some age on me: Social organization of older people in a rural American community.* Lexington: University Press of Kentucky.

Weiss, R. S. (1973). *Loneliness: The experience of emotional and social isolation.* Cambridge: MIT Press.

Weiss, R. S. (1989). Reflections on the present state of loneliness research. In M. Hojat & R. Crandall (Eds.), *Loneliness: Theory, research, and applications* (pp. 1–16). Newbury Park, CA: Sage.

Wellman, B. (1981). Applying network analysis to the study of support. In B. H. Gottlieb (Ed.), *Social networks and social support* (pp. 171–200). Beverly Hills, CA: Sage.

Wellman, B., & Leighton, B. (1979). Networks, neighborhoods and communities. *Urban Affairs Quarterly, 15,* 363–390.

Wenger, G. C. (1989). Support networks in old age: Constructing a typology. In M. Jefferys (Ed.), *Growing old in the twentieth century.* London: Routledge.

Yarcheski, A., Scolovino, M. A., & Mahon, N. E. (1994). Social support and well-being in adolescents: The mediating role of hopefulness. *Nursing Research, 43,* 288–292.

Yates, B. C. (1995). The relationships between social support and short- and long-term recovery outcomes in men with coronary heart disease. *Research in Nursing & Health, 18,* 193–203.

CHAPTER 7

Qualitative Research and Chronic Illness

Janice M. Morse* and Cheryl A. Dellasega

While most older adults have at least one if not more functional impairments, the type and degree of the individual incapacity varies greatly. For example, the leading functional disability among older adults is mobility impairment (U.S. Bureau of the Census, 1992); yet there are great qualitative differences between the lifestyles of persons who are so crippled with arthritis that they cannot move from the home environment and those who experience discomfort when ambulating up and down steps but do not become homebound.

Individual variations in health status and the accumulation of diverse life experiences make a linear perspective of the life situation of older persons inappropriate (Ford, 1987). Although our understanding of the aging process is based primarily on the generalized experiences of older persons who have lived through the Great Depression and two major world wars, this perspective may soon be outdated. The current generation of elders who take an active interest in health promotion (Schafer, 1989) and wellness are likely to redefine what we are willing to accept as illness and how health is defined in the later years.

However, even if the level of acceptable disability associated with aging changes, the types of problems that afflict older adults, which are primarily chronic in nature, are not likely to be altered. Heart disease, malignant neoplasms, cerebrovascular disease, chronic obstructive pulmonary disease,

*Address correspondence to Dr. C. Dellasega, School of Nursing, The Pennsylvania State University, University Park, PA 16801; the telephone number is (814) 863-2224, and fax number is (814) 863-3779.

atherosclerosis, and diabetes mellitus are chronic conditions that have consistently been the leading causes of death among persons aged 65 and over in the last decades (Brody, Brock, & Williams, 1987). Each of these problems requires a different type of physiologic and psychologic coping than acute health problems.

Chronic illness is defined as "an altered health state that will not be cured by a simple surgical procedure or a short course of medical therapy" (Fitzgerald, 1992, p. 4). Fitzgerald points out two unique aspects of chronic illness: (1) the multiple incapacities that often result and (2) the knowledge that the individual will never completely recover from the condition. Consequently, special demands for coping are placed on both the individual and his or her family when this type of illness occurs.

The patient tasks associated with learning to live with a chronic illness include (1) acclimating to a lack of privacy, (2) being willing to share information about intimate body functions, (3) living with constant scrutiny into one's lifestyle, and (4) assuming responsibility for self-monitoring (Fitzgerald, 1992). Family members, meanwhile, must develop skills to assist and support the patient with implementation of daily therapies.

In addition to dealing with difficulties associated with chronic illness, the aging person is confronted with developmental tasks, many of which relate to transcending physical problems (Reed, 1991). Psychological responses to aging, in addition to grieving over lost functions, can occur in both the individual and his or her family (Duvall, 1967). Two prominent developmental theorists, Peck (1968) and Havinghurst (1952), specify that coping with physical changes of aging, including loss of function, is an important developmental task during the later years. For instance, over half of all elderly persons suffer from some degree of degenerative joint disease (Cohen & Van Nostrand, 1994), which can limit their ability to remain independent. This results in the elders having to modify their lifestyles to compensate for these deficits and needing to cope psychologically with the loss of mobility. Furthermore, the older person's family must also adjust to the older person's loss of independence as, for example, when he or she becomes dependent on the family members for many activities of daily living, such as shopping, bathing, meal preparation, and administering medicine.

A comprehensive understanding of chronic illness and its impact on the life situation of an older adult is needed to appreciate fully the aging experience. Unidimensional, deductive, quantitative approaches that have emerged from the positivist/empiricist paradigm fail to capture the full context of life for an elderly person with chronic illness. For instance, as Carter, Elward, Malmgren, Martin, and Larson (1991) point out, survey research with older subjects is more likely to be biased because elders are more heterogeneous and should not be considered a uniform group. Phillips (1989) also criticizes research that takes into account "phenomenon stability in relation to age" (p. 182), suggesting that great differences exist among older individuals.

Qualitative strategies offer a richer understanding of individual experience and are especially appropriate for studies of the chronically ill elderly. When chronic illness is introduced as a variable in addition to age, it becomes even more important to consider individualized approaches, such as those that are offered by qualitative approaches. As stated by Wilson (1993), "Naturalistic approaches are based on a conviction that to know *about* people is not enough" (p. 5).

It is also important to note that the various methods available through qualitative strategies offer a more in-depth exploration of many issues related to disability and aging. Naturalistic inquiry enables the researcher to examine the elder's experience from his or her own perspective and consider context in the process of inquiry, enables the researcher to account for individual variations in the development of models and theory, and provides a mechanism for exploring phenomena about which little is known.

The purpose of this chapter is to describe first how qualitative methods must be modified when conducting research with elders and, second, to discuss the contribution of qualitative research to understanding the phenomenon of chronic illness in older adults.

CONDUCTING QUALITATIVE RESEARCH WITH OLDER ADULTS

The aging process places some constraints on the conduct of qualitative research with elderly participants. For example, as participants are interviewed, special consideration must be made and the normal interview process adapted. In addition, when conducting research with special subgroups of elderly persons, such as an Alzheimer's patient, research methods must be selected with respect to limitations imposed on subjects by the disease.

In this section, we will describe the special conditions occurring as a consequence of the aging process and diseases that primarily affect elders.

Strategies for modifying or selecting qualitative methods to address these conditions will be presented.

Designing the Study

Physical restrictions secondary to aging, which can affect the "old-old" (age 85+) in particular, can make many forms of data collection difficult, if not impossible. For instance, failing eyesight may make the use of written forms of data collection, such as semistructured questions, infeasible because elders, even with large print forms, may not be able to read the questions. As elders overall have lower educational levels, literacy may be a problem, which may be a special concern for minority groups, where facility with the English language may further compound problems with reading. Furthermore, arthritis may restrict the ability of elders to hold a pencil and write answers on the questionnaire. Therefore, certain forms of data collection are more suited to elders than others and should be considered when designing the study.

While questionnaires, or even semistructured questionnaires, may be administered to some elderly populations, unstructured tape-recorded interviews may be more suitable for data collection. Such a decision would change the research from a quantitative design to narrative inquiry, providing the questions could still be answered. With cognitively impaired samples, the use of interviews may not be feasible, and the researcher is restricted to collect data using participant observations or videotaped data. Hurley, Volicer, Hanrahan, Houde, and Volicer (1992) used an innovative approach by interviewing nurses who worked closely with Alzheimer's patients and then structuring a pain assessment tool from their responses.

These issues are significant when planning the research, for the quality of the investigation and the match between the research question and the data collected may be irrevocably altered if the wrong methods are selected. This mismatch may be a major threat to the validity of the study—the researcher should consider, prior to data collection, what types of data will be obtained using this less than optimal method. It may be possible that the questions may have to be changed slightly, the focus of the study altered, a different sample used, or the study abandoned altogether. The research should proactively consider the potential abilities (and disabilities) of the elderly participants in the study during the proposal stage. For instance, deciding in advance to exclude all cognitively impaired participants, a common practice among gerontologic researchers, may result in the exclusion of 80% of the study population. It is preferable for the investigator to select a method that permits cognitively impaired persons to be included.

Obtaining Consent

If the elderly participant is oriented and cognitively intact, then informed consent may be obtained according to usual protocol. Difficulties arise, however, when the elderly participant is confused or unable to comprehend the purposes of the study, what would be involved, and the significance of the consent procedure itself. Many elders also prefer to defer decision making to a family member, even if they are capable of doing so themselves (Kapp, 1991).

Kayser-Jones and Koenig (1994) note that the voluntariness of consent may be jeopardized by the elderly person's "desire for human contact (even with a researcher) as a result of social isolation" or from a feeling of coercion (p. 19). The elder may also participate without fully comprehending the nature and the purpose of the research study. Despite the fact that consent is negotiated prior to the beginning of data collection, Kayser-Jones and Koenig note that the researcher must "engage in an almost daily process of obtaining 'informal informed consent', constantly re-explaining the purpose and the requirements of the study" (p. 20).

In some regions, regulations have been established to guide researchers through this process. The participant's next of kin may legally provide consent, so that the patient's spouse or child may be approached to provide consent on the participant's behalf. However, in other locations (e.g., in Alberta, Canada), the elderly confused become wards, under the Dependent Adult Act, which states that the next of kin must make application to the agency to retain guardianship. Such regulations actually assist the researcher to get permission, as, for example, in cases where the potential participant does not have relatives. Of course, if relatives are available but have not applied for guardianship, it is still wise to obtain additional permissions from them, even if they cannot legally provide consent. Likewise, the elderly participant should always be asked for consent, in addition to his or her legal guardian, to promote cooperation and to ensure that all institutional requirements governing access to residents are met. The bottom line is that it is the responsibility of the researcher to ascertain if such regulations are in effect in the area where the research is to be carried out.

Despite the establishment of standardized regulations, Drane (1984) presents a model for assessing the elder's competency to provide consent based on the patient's capacity to choose. Drane's preference, which is individualized and flexible, must supplement consents obtained from participants' guardians. Although Drane's model was developed for the obtaining of informed consent for *treatment*, it is equally useful for obtaining consent for participation in research.

While Drane's model is based on three levels of consent depending on the risks inherent in treatment protocol, qualitative research is generally considered low risk, so only the first level of assessment will be presented here. Drane's (1984) *Standard I* is for use with low-risk situations and when the participant is confused but has some level of awareness. "Such terms as *'virtually competent, marginally competent*, and *competent for practical purposes'*" (p. 2) may be applied to these potential participants. In this case, *assessment* should be obtained from the participant. The participant should be given an appropriate explanation about the research project, and if the potential participant objects, that participant's wishes must be respected by the researcher and that person must be excluded from the sample regardless of the consent obtained from the elder's guardian.

Qualitative research conducted with elders is not always covered under the rubric *expedited review.* While the procedures themselves are not likely to cause physical harm to elders, the research question(s) that qualitative researchers are interested in may place the elderly participants at risk. For instance, exploring the behavioral effects of removing restraints (Morse & McHutchion, 1991) involved collecting data by continuously videotaping the participant for 1 week with the restraints on and 1 week with the restraints off. These surveillance procedures reduced the possibility that injury may occur from a fall, although the cameras were situated so that if personal care was being provided and curtains were pulled around the bed to obscure the view of the camera, there was still the concern that collecting videotaped data posed a risk of invasion of privacy to the participant. Thus research of this nature would be subject to full review by the ethics committee for the careful weighing of the risks and benefits of the research, prior to giving approval.

Following the principles of all research, the explanation provided to participants must be targeted to their educational level and level of comprehension. The consent form should be constructed with consideration for the limitations of aging, such as printing the consent form with large type. Remember, even if the patient is cognitively impaired and has not officially given his or her own consent for the study, the principles of ongoing consent still remain. The onus is on the researcher to frequently remind the participants why they are there and of the purpose of the study. If the participant indicates that he or she does not want the researcher present, then the researcher must leave.

Collecting Data

When conducting research with elders, all the standard principles for collecting and managing data apply. However, there are a few pitfalls that should be considered in the process of interviewing or conducting participant observation.

Interviewing

When conducting an open-ended interview, there are some areas that need special consideration. As an unstructured, interactive interview often takes more than 1 hour, it is important that the elderly person be seated comfortably, be free from discomfort secondary to pain or a full bladder, and be warm. The quality of the recording equipment is important, and some technical aspects also need to be considered because the elderly person may have a dry mouth or loose dentures, which would impair recording. An excellent external microphone that will pick up the participant's voice, even if faint, is essential. This is important, for if the quality of the recording is poor or inaudible, the inability to hear the tape slows the process of transcription (therefore increasing the cost) and may result in missing words or even blocks of text.

Many elders appreciate the opportunity for conversation, especially if there is an attentive listener; yet collecting narratives is not without difficulties. Sometimes, the participant's stories will have little apparent relevance to the research question, and the participant may seem to ramble, making it difficult to obtain the anticipated information. Hearing impairments may make the interview process itself difficult. Ensure that if the elderly participant uses a hearing aid, it is worn and functions. Otherwise, make sure that he or she has heard and understood the interview question. If the researcher suspects that the participant tends to forget the questions, frequent reminders, even interruptions, may be necessary. It may be helpful to have the subject follow the spoken questions with an identical printed version that he or she can hold. At all times observe the participant for signs of fatigue, giving him or her breaks when needed, and terminate the interview if necessary. West, Bondy, and Hutchinson (1991) note that limitations from interviewing elders may be overcome by increasing the sample size, returning to the site frequently to obtain adequate data, lengthening the observational periods, recognizing the value of stories, adding participant observation components, and using videotapes.

Observational methods are gaining increasing importance with the cognitively impaired. The participant's impairment may mean that the participant is unaware of the observer, thereby reducing interactive effects, or the confused elder may become anxious, wondering why someone is hovering about his or her room. A sensitive assessment of each situation by the observer is necessary, and preliminary pilot work to circumvent these problems is important.

Data Analysis

Data from these studies are managed according to the techniques of all qualitative data. However, when analyzing these data, as with all data, it is important to consider the context in which the data were obtained. This consideration is always from the *emic* perspective, that is, from the perspective of the participant (Luborsky, 1994, p. 190). These collected data are a life history, so each period should be interpreted according to the period in which it was referred. Context is also important to include. For example, nursing home data must be interpreted according to the values, beliefs, and norms of the nursing home itself.

If the research methods selected require that the emerging theory be confirmed with the participants (e.g., as with the case with grounded theory), then, if possible, this should be done. If it is not possible, then it is permissible to confirm the findings with a secondary sample. For example, the nurses caring for the participants or family members could be used. At all times, the researcher must select these secondary participants with the awareness that the information obtained from the primary participants was obtained with assurances of anonymity and confidentiality. Presenting the theory for confirmation must be done, therefore, in such a manner that individual participants cannot be identified.

QUALITATIVE RESEARCH AND THE CHRONICALLY ILL ELDERLY

In this section, the contribution of qualitative research to the understanding of the phenomena of chronic illness in the older adult will be presented.

First, a description of the illness *experience* of the elder will be presented, and second, studies that address the inclusion of environmental context in our understanding of illness (i.e., living at home with a disability or nursing home studies) will be reviewed. Third, studies that address the caregiving relationship for the elderly patient will be presented, in particular, caregiving for the patient with Alzheimer's Disease. Finally, studies that provide a more comprehensive understanding of the experience will be addressed. For instance, studies that reveal the experience of transitions (such as the transition of admission to a nursing home) or changes that occur over time with the chronically ill elderly will be discussed.

The Illness Experience in Older Adults

Surprisingly, there are relatively few qualitative studies of elders themselves and their experiences of illness. This may be due, in part, to the difficulties mentioned in conducting research with this population. However, those researchers who have investigated illness using elders as participants have conducted very interesting and important research. For instance, Haggstrom, Axelsson, and Norberg (1994) attempted the ambitious task of eliciting the experience of living with a stroke. Their study used a projective technique—using photographs of an elderly person being fed or eating independently—and asked the participants to discuss the photographs. Several themes emerged: uncertainty, sadness, and mourning; gratefulness, hope, and satisfaction; and isolation. The authors stressed that the metaphor and stories related by the elders provided caregivers with the language and information *essential* for the provision of empathetic care and essential for assisting the patients to move on, "to find their own voices, and to take charge of their own histories" (p. 335).

The subjective experience of forgetfulness was explored by Cromwell (1994) using grounded theory. Cromwell identified first the perceived loss of and attempts to regain "identity continuity and personal competence" (p. 449). By understanding the process of coping of those residents who were striving to "continue to be who I am," important strategies to assist elders who have memory problems were identified. These included ways to help elders improve their self-esteem, the development of "new role scripts" to facilitate the continuance of values roles, and teaching the elders new strategies of coping with forgetting. A significant feature of both of these studies is the important recommendations that the authors have for improving practice. Qualitative research frequently produces pragmatic and obvious outcomes that may be implemented immediately to improve care.

The Exploration of Context

The Environmental Context

An important aspect of both chronic illness and aging is the environment in which the elder is situated. In this area, a disproportionately large number of studies biased toward the institutional setting have been conducted. Although the presence of a chronic illness does not directly predict that the older adult will reside in a nursing home, increasing disability in conjunction with lack of social support do make institutionalization more likely. However, other settings, such as the hospital and home, should not be overlooked.

Living at Home

Over 90% of older persons, including most of the chronically ill, live at home (U.S. Bureau of the Census, 1992). Study of older persons in the home setting is often difficult due to problems with access; however, such studies are critical. As elders become increasingly incapacitated, they become more dependent on their spouses, on their social network, and on social services (such as "Meals-on-Wheels," home care, and visiting nurses). As their spouses are likely to be in the same age range (and therefore likely also to be suffering from a chronic illness or disability), these couples may not be able to care for each other. With increased isolation, the loss of independence and loss of personal control occur in the homebound population, similar to those residents in the institutional setting (Folden, 1990). An in-depth exploration of this dynamic would be an appropriate strategy for qualitative researchers.

The role of others in the environment is another perspective that lends itself to qualitative strategies. As wives statistically outlive their husbands, neighborhoods tend to have disproportionately large numbers of widows living alone. The caregiving responsibility frequently falls on the unmarried daughter, and many qualitative studies have recently examined the experiences of middle-aged daughters caring for their aged mother in the home (Lynch-Sauer, 1990; Opie, 1994; Thibodeau, 1993). Most of these studies have used some form of interview method, focusing on the experience of being cared for at home, or, if the elder has Alzheimer's or some illness that makes interviewing difficult, then the caregivers themselves were interviewed.

These studies have been important, providing insights that could not be obtained from quantitative approaches. For instance, Abel (1991) observed that prior to the onset of Alzheimer's, daughters considered that their main goal in caregiving was to protect their parents' autonomy. As the dementia progressed, daughters protected their mothers' dignity by "pretending that nothing had changed," including preventing them from realizing that they had lost control of the decisions in their lives, and thus preserving their sense of uniqueness and competence.

Qualitative research can also add important insights into the difficulties and dangers of living alone (such as falling, loneliness, the need for obtaining adequate nutrition and hygiene, and caregiver burden and burnout), offering a more complete understanding of the phenomenon or even a means for identifying a solution.

Living in a Nursing Home

While several types of institutions are available to offer different levels of support for chronically ill elderly, each requires different degrees of adjustment for older persons who are admitted. For example, personal care boarding homes, day care centers, and continuing care retirement centers all offer different amounts of structure. Unfortunately, most of the studies have been conducted in nursing homes, and there are few studies of the homebound elderly or those in the acute care setting. Qualitative studies conducted in nursing home settings have primarily used the ethnographic methods. A classical study, *Living and dying at Murray Manor* (Gubrium, 1973), has been most influential in this area.

Ethnography provides a detailed and rich description of the day-to-day lives of those in the nursing home, thus bringing otherwise silent issues to public awareness. Issues such as patient noncommunication, the rote routine of care, the lack of resident privacy, control, and dignity can be presented and explored. An ambitious cross-cultural study comparing a nursing home in Scotland with one in the United States (Kayser-Jones, 1981) revealed that many of the nursing home conditions were a direct result of the staff's philosophy of care, rather than resulting from patient needs per se. For instance, that the use of restraints was not a universal requisite for the provision of safe care was a surprising and significant finding. Likewise, the passivity of residents and their ability to obtain favors from staff varied greatly between the two institutions, and this factor had important ramifications for the well-being of residents.

In a creative project, Hymen, Bulkin, and Woog (1993) explored the *staff's* perception of the nursing home. They uncovered a tension between the staff's vocation to *care* and the institution's need for efficiency. Paradoxically, at the same time they found, among other things, a "lack of caring ethos implicit in the staff's relative silence about death and dying" (p. 209). Such careful analysis of conflicting values provides important clues into staff frustrations, working conditions, and the environment of the nursing home.

Exploring the Acute Care Setting

Differing from the nursing home in both the severity of the illness and the length of stay, the acute care setting and the care of elders have not been extensively examined using qualitative approaches. Fisher and Peterson (1993) examined the operating room staff's attitudes toward the elderly client. They found that the surgeon had little respect for elders, and these attitudes greatly influenced the quality of care provided. Because of the imbalance of power between surgeons and nurses, nurses were silent about the compromised care and treatment of elders.

Qualitative methods can also provide the techniques for microanalysis. For example, communication patterns can be explored using these techniques. In a study of communication competence of elders during admission to an acute care setting, Van Cott (1993) found that the elderly person's misperception of speech resulted in a source of conflict in the nurse-patient relationship. When conducting a nursing assessment, the nurse's agenda was to complete the form. The elderly patient, on the other hand, was intent on establishing a relationship with the nurse and answered her questions with an "indirect narrative." The elderly patients tended to express their concerns with "apparently irrelevant stories," and analyses of these dialogues revealed that psychosocial aspects of care were not addressed.

Family and Support Networks

In the home setting, caregiving by a spouse or family member is a vital component of the support network for older adults. In this topical area, studies that offer perspectives on relationships between chronically ill elders and their significant others have tended to use qualitative strategies. A study published in the first issue of *Nursing Research* reports on interviews of family caregivers conducted by Mack (1952). More recently, a review of nursing studies about older adults showed that half of the investigations reported used qualitative strategies to explore family caregiving relationships (Lang, Kraegel, Rantz, & Krejci, 1990).

Caregiving issues are especially relevant for older persons with chronic mental illness, such as dementia. Although numerous studies on this subject have been conducted using quantitative approaches, qualitative strategies have recently been implemented that enhance the findings of previous studies. Literature reviews of gerontological studies conducted in 1983 by Wolanin and in 1986 by Adams documented that the majority of studies at both time periods focused on prevalence rates. More recently, two qualitative studies by Collins, Liken, King, and Kokinakis (1993) and Jones and Martinson (1992) offered insight on themes of loss experienced by family caregivers after bereavement that would not have been uncovered with quantitative types of research.

Finally, using focus groups to explore the physician-caregiver relationship in Alzheimer's Disease, Morgan and Zhao (1993) found that physicians referred to elders in a negative manner more frequently than in a positive one. Furthermore, caregivers were also negative when discussing their physicians and had a negative attitude toward medical and nonmedical advice. The authors attribute this breakdown in relationships to the emotional issues that the caregivers were forced to confront. The caregivers' difficulty in dealing with these issues "carried over" into the doctor-caregiver relationship.

Another application of qualitative research is to the structure of nursing practice itself. Numerous studies have examined caring actions and professional relationships. For instance, Tagliareni, Mengel, and Sherman (1993) used focus groups to tease out differences between gerontological nursing practice in acute and long-term care settings.

The Experience of Change

Qualitative studies have enhanced the understanding of transitional stages in an elder's life. For example, in her qualitative study of new admissions to a skilled care facility, Chenitz (1980) found that elderly persons often rationalized their admission to the facility. Dellasega and Mastrian (1995) found that even family members experienced an adjustment period after the placement of their loved one in a skilled care facility.

In a longitudinal study, Willoughby and Keating (1991) developed a five-stage model of relinquishing the control of caregiving. The stages identified were:

1. emerging recognition of the Alzheimer's;
2. taking control (in which caregiver is isolated and does not receive much help from outside);
3. losing control and accepting the decision of others to admit to an institution;
4. adjusting to the psychiatric institutions; and
5. after recognizing the loss of the relative, moving on and resuming one's own life.

These insights into the dynamics of the change process reflect the utility and strength of qualitative studies.

APPLICATION OF QUALITATIVE RESEARCH TO CARE OF OLDER ADULTS

Application to Knowledge Development

In this section, the contribution of qualitative research to gerontological knowledge will be discussed. The section is organized according to the levels of qualitative research, from descriptive research to interpretive; to concept development; and to theory development.

Descriptive research

While lay descriptions of illness may not be considered a form of qualitative research, many poignant writings emerge from the lay literature providing important details about the lives of elders. For instance, Seaver's (1994) description of residence in an institution titled "My world now: Life in a nursing home, from the inside" appeared in *Newsweek* and attracted much comment. Similar pieces published in the *New York Times* and other newspapers and magazines, as well as May Sarton's epic novel *As we are now,* also have received a great deal of attention. Provided these writings are considered valid, they may be used by the qualitative researcher *as data,* an approach adopted by Lynch-Sauer (1990). Alternatively, lay descriptions may be considered a source for potential research questions.

Descriptive research literature, even if the description is from a single case, differs from lay descriptions in two important ways. First, these descriptions have been validated or confirmed, and second, these data have been analyzed and placed in the context of current theory and literature. Of course, the description may be derived from several events or participants, so that the results are a synthesis of these experiences, thus forming an even richer, thick description.

There have been several descriptive studies using observational methods, including videotape. For instance, observational studies of the behavior of Alzheimer's patients provide important information, especially when the patients are so cognitively impaired that they cannot be interviewed. As a part of a larger quantitative project on patient falls, Morse, Tylko, and Dixon (1987), noted that the way that patients move about the room and the placement of furniture were important factors in fall prevention. Whereas previous recommendations had been to remove furniture from the patients' rooms, so that if patients fell, they would not hurt themselves further by falling on furniture, Morse et al. observed that patients with an impaired gait moved about the room by "island hopping," that is, by grasping furniture to maintain balance if they did not have a suitable walking aid. So important was this feature that the placement of the furniture dictated their route from the bed to the bathroom, and if there was not a direct route, then patients "dove" from one furniture handhold to the next. Thus clinically, for those who did not use walking aids but rather moved about, island hopping, a sensible nursing strategy would be to "build a path" of conveniently high objects that would provide secure support for the patients to get to the bathroom.

Concept Development

Research at the conceptual level with aging and elders has been sparse but is gaining significance. This type of research provides crucial information that must necessarily precede theory development. For instance, in a study of privacy within a nursing home, Applegate and Morse (1994) noted that there were three types of relationships: between staff and patient, between patients and patients, and between patients and staff. They could treat one another as a friend, as a stranger, or as an object. When these data were compared with data on the type of relationship between dyads, where violations of the privacy occurred, all the violations to privacy occurred within interactions in which people treated one another as an object. When the participants treated each other as strangers, the relationship was cordial; when they treated each other as friends, the relationship was intimate, and there was an exchange of favors. In both of these cases, privacy was respected.

Theory Development

Despite the fact that there are several theories describing the chronic illness experience (Corbin & Strauss, 1991; Morse & Johnson, 1993; Robinson, 1993; Thorne, 1992), and while all of these theories *may* be applicable to elders with chronic illness, none were developed specifically from the experience of the elderly client. Note that we have only suggested that these theories *may* be applicable—in fact, these theories have not been applied to elderly client populations. For instance, Robinson's theory of *normalization* in families was developed from a pediatric population. The basic tenet, that families with a chronically ill child work toward normalizing the illness experience, may be only partly true for elders. A case in point is Abel's (1991) study of daughters of Alzheimer's patients; initially daughters did try to normalize and cover the illness. However, as the elderly parent continued to decline, there came a point when it was no longer possible to continue to normalize, and the realities of the disease had to be faced. Continued deterioration is not a part of the theory of normalization, but rather relative stabilization of the chronicity. Therefore, in addition to developing theories of illness from the illness experience of elders, existing theories must be tested for fit with this population, prior to application.

Nevertheless, one of these theories has been operationalized for elderly clients with chronic illness (Robinson et al., 1993)—that is the Corbin and Strauss Illness Trajectory Framework (1991). In a proposal, these authors identified eight phase-specific protocols and published two of these protocols for the *pretrajectory phase* and the *unstable phase.* This work has important applications that make the model useful in the clinical setting, and it is clear that much similar work needs to be done with all of these models.

CONCLUSION

The ANA Standards of Gerontologic Nursing Practice (American Nurses Association, 1988) guide the practice of nurses who work with older adults.

The contribution of qualitative research to practice can be seen in relation to several of these standards but is most relevant to standard No. 2 ("The nurse participates in the generation and testing of theory as a basis for clinical decisions") and to standard No. 9 ("The nurse participates in research designed to generate an organized body of gerontological nursing knowledge, disseminates research findings, and uses them in practice").

As pointed out by Wilson (1993), in clinical nursing practice, qualitative approaches to problems are common because gerontological nurses rely primarily on subjective information to assess and intervene with their patients. Wilson also noted that the positivist approach tells us the "that"—only that a certain condition is present—while naturalistic techniques describe the "how." It is the "how" that is often most relevant to clinical practice. Qualitative research takes research beyond the "either/or, more/less, yes/no levels of analysis" (Gubrium, 1993). Qualitative methods provide a means to develop valid explanations, to identify and describe concepts, and to develop valid theories. It is evident that qualitative inquiry has made and will continue to make a significant contribution to gerontological research.

REFERENCES

Abel, E. K. (1991). *Who cares for the elderly? Public policy and the experiences of adult daughters.* Philadelphia: Temple University Press.

Adams, M. (1986). Aging: Gerontological nursing research. In H. Werley, J. Fitzpatrick, & R. Taunton (Eds.), *Annual review of nursing research* (pp. 77–103). New York: Springer.

American Nurses Association. (1988). *Scope and standards of gerontologic nursing practice.* Kansas City, MO: Author.

Applegate, M., & Morse, J. M. (1994). Personal privacy and interactional patterns in a nursing home. *Journal of Aging Studies, 8*(4), 413–434.

Brody, J., Brock, D., & Williams, T. (1987). Trends in the health of the elderly population. *Annual Review of Public Health, 8,* 211–234.

Carter, W., Elward, K., Malmgren, J., Martin, M., & Larson, E. (1991). Participation of older adults in health programs and research: A critical review of the literature. *Gerontologist, 31*(5), 584–592.

Chenitz, W. C. (1980). Adjusting to institutional life: Status passage for the aged. *Gerontologist, 20*(5), 80.

Cohen, R., & Van Nostrand, J. (1994). *Highlights of trends in the health of older Americans: United States, 1994.* Washington, DC: U.S. Department of Health and Human Services.

Collins, C., Liken, M., King, S., & Kokinakis, C. (1993). Loss and grief among family caregivers of relatives with dementia. *Qualitative Health Research, 3*(2), 236–253.

Corbin, J., & Strauss, A. (1991). A nursing model for chronic illness management based upon the Illness Trajectory Framework. *Scholarly Inquiry for Nursing Practice, 5*(3), 155–174.

Cromwell, S. L. (1994). The subjective experience of forgetfulness among elders. *Qualitative Health Research, 4*(4), 444–462.

Dellasega, C., & Mastrian, K. (1995). The process and consequences of institutionalizing an elder. *Western Journal of Nursing Research, 17*(2), 123–137.

Drane, J. F. (1984). Competency to give an informed consent: A model for making clinical assessments. *Journal of the American Medical Association, 252*(2), 925–927.

Duvall, E. (1967). *Family development* (3rd ed.). Philadelphia: J. B. Lippincott.

Fisher, B. J., & Peterson, C. (1993). "She won't be dancing much anyway": A study of surgeons, surgical nurses, and elderly patients. *Qualitative Health Research, 3*(2), 165–183.

Fitzgerald, J. (1992). *Coping with chronic illness: Overcoming powerlessness* (2nd ed.). Philadelphia: F. A. Davis.

Folden, S. (1990). On the inside looking out: Perceptions of the homebound. *Journal of Gerontological Nursing, 16*(1), 9–15.

Ford, D. (1987). *Humans as self-constructing living systems: A developmental perspective on behavior and personality.* Hillsdale, NJ: Erlbaum.

Gubrium, J. (1973). *Living and dying at Murray Manor.* New York: St. Martin's Press.

Gubrium, J. (1993). Contributions of qualitative research to aging [Editorial]. *Qualitative Health Research, 3*(2), 131–132.

Haggstrom, T, Axelsson, K., & Norberg, A. (1994). The experience of living with stroke sequelae illuminated by means of stories and metaphors. *Qualitative Health Research, 4*(3), 321–337.

Havinghurst, R. (1952). *Developmental tasks and education.* New York: David McKay.

Hurley, A., Volicer, B., Hanrahan, P., Houde, S., & Volicer, L. (1992). Assessment of discomfort in advanced Alzheimer patients. *Research in Nursing & Health, 15,* 369–377.

Hyman, R. B., Bulkin, W., & Woog, P. C. (1993). The staff's perception of a skilled nursing facility. *Qualitative Health Research, 3*(2), 209–235.

Jones, P., & Martinson, I. (1992). The experience of bereavement in caregivers of family members with Alzheimer's disease. *Image: Journal of Nursing Scholarship, 24*(3), 172–176.

Kapp, M. (1991). Health care decision-making by the elderly: I get by with a little help from my family. *Gerontologist, 31*(5), 619–623.

Kayser-Jones. J. (1981). *Old, alone, and neglected: Care of the aged in Scotland and the United States.* Berkeley: University of California Press.

Kayser-Jones, J., & Koenig, B. A. (1994). Ethical issues. In J. Gubrium & A. Sankar (Eds.), *Qualitative methods in aging research* (pp. 15–32). Thousand Oaks, CA: Sage.

Lang, N., Kraegel, J., Rantz, M., & Krejci, J. (1990). *Quality of health care for older people in America: A review of nursing studies.* Kansas City, MO: American Nurses Association.

Luborsky, M. R. (1994) The identification of themes and patterns. In J. Gubrium & A. Sankar (Eds.), *Qualitative methods in aging research* (pp. 189–210). Thousand Oaks, CA: Sage.

Lynch-Sauer, J. (1990). When a family member has Alzheimer's Disease: A phenomenological description of caregiving. *Journal of Gerontological Nursing, 16*(9), 8–11.

Mack, M. (1952). The personal adjustment of chronically ill old people under home care. *Nursing Research, 1*(1), 9–30.

Morgan, D. L., & Zhao, P. Z. (1993). The doctor-caregiver relationship: Managing care of family members with Alzheimer's disease. *Qualitative Health Research, 3*(2), 133–164.

Morse, J. M., & Johnson, J. (1993). Toward a theory of illness: The illness constellation model. In J. M. Morse & J. L. Johnson (Eds.), *The illness experience: Dimensions of suffering* (pp. 315–342). Newbury Park, CA: Sage.

Morse, J. M., & McHutchion, E. (1991). The behavioral effects of releasing restraints. *Research in Nursing and Health, 14,* 187–196.

Morse, J. M., Tylko, S., & Dixon, H. A. (1987). Characteristics of patients that fall. *Gerontologist, 27*(4), 516–522.

Opie, A. (1994). The instability of the caring body: Gender and caregivers of confused older people. *Qualitative Health Research, 4*(1), 31–50.

Peck, R. (1968). Psychological developments in the second half of life. In B. L. Neugarten (Ed.), *Middle age and aging* (p. 88). Chicago: University of Chicago Press.

Phillips, L. (1989). Age: A truly confounding variable. *Western Journal of Nursing Research, 11*(2), 181–195.

Reed, P. (1991). Toward a nursing theory of self-transcendence: Deductive reformulation using developmental theories. *Advances in Nursing Science, 13*(4), 64–77.

Robinson, C. (1993). Managing life with a chronic condition: The story of normalization. *Qualitative Health Research, 3*(1), 6–28.

Robinson, L., Bevil, C., Arcangelo, V., Reifsnyder, J., Rothman, N., & Smeltzer, S. (1993). Operationalizing the Corbin and Strauss Trajectory Model for elderly clients with chronic illness. *Scholarly Inquiry for Nursing Practice, 7*(4), 253–264.

Schafer, S. (1989). Aggressive approach to promoting health responsibility. *Journal of Gerontological Nursing, 15*(22).

Seaver, A. (1994, June 27). My world now: Life in a nursing home, from the inside. *Newsweek, CXXIII*(26), 11.

Tagliareni, E., Mengel, A., & Sherman, S. (1993). Parallel worlds of nursing practice. In M. Burke & S. Sherman (Eds.), *Ways of knowing and caring for older adults* (pp. 91–106). New York: NLN Press.

Thibodeau, J. (1993, Jan-Feb). Caring for a parent: A phenomenologic inquiry. *Nursing Outlook, 41*(1), 15–19.

Thorne, S. (1992). *Negotiating health care: The social context of illness.* Newbury Park, CA: Sage.

U.S. Bureau of the Census. (1992). *Current Population Reports, Special Studies, P23–178RV, Sixty-five plus in America.* Washington, DC: U.S. Government Printing Office.

Van Cott, M. L. (1993). Communicative competence during nursing admission interviews of elderly patients in acute care settings. *Qualitative Health Research, 3*(2), 184–208.

West, M., Bondy, E., & Hutchinson, S. (1991). Interviewing institutionalized elders: Threats to validity. *Image: Journal of Nursing Scholarship, 23,* 171–176.

Willoughby, J., & Keating, N. (1991). Being in control: The process of caring for a relative with Alzheimer's disease. *Qualitative Health Research, 1*(1), 27–50.

Wilson, H. (1993). Ways of knowing: Shaping the chaos. In M. Burke & S. Sherman (Eds.), *Ways of knowing and caring for older adults* (pp. 1–16). New York: NLN Press.

Wolanin, M. (1983). Clinical geriatric nursing research. In H. Werley & J. Fitzpatrick (Eds.), *Annual review of nursing research* (pp. 75–97). New York: Springer.

CHAPTER 8

Nursing Homes and the Chronically Ill Resident: Policy and Issues

Marilyn J. Rantz and
Mary Zwygart-Stauffacher

In no other health care arena have policy and governmental regulations been used as much to influence services than in the institutions that provide long-term care to residents who are chronically ill. Historically, controversy surrounds the issue of whether nursing homes in America are providing good or poor quality care; consistently, the official governmental response to concerns about quality has been various kinds of policy initiatives in the form of governmental regulations (Kane, 1988). There are licensure, certification, inspection of care, and regulation of nursing and nursing home personnel, as well as ombudsman programs organized under the Older Americans Act. Despite these efforts initiated in the 1970s and early 1980s, quality problems in nursing homes continue (Kane). Policy initiatives continue as well.

Zimmerman (1991) summarized the policy milestones for long-term care beginning with the Health Care Financing Administration's (HCFA) commissioning a major review of quality of care in nursing homes by the Institute of Medicine (IOM) in 1983. The 1986 IOM report culminated in legislative mandates of the Omnibus Budget Reconciliation Act of 1987 (OBRA 87), which was implemented in October 1990. This legislation stimulated sweeping changes in long-term care. The legislative effort heavily focused on (1) determining effective patient outcomes, (2) establishing quality assurance programs within each facility, (3) carefully assessing individual resident needs, (4) improving the educational base of the nonprofessional staff, and (5) increasing the numbers of professional staff working in long-term care facilities (Migdail, 1992).

Policy initiatives must be put in perspective. The nursing home industry is a major provider of health care services. There are over 27,000 nursing homes in the United States; 75% are privately owned, for-profit facilities. Since the 1960s, there has been a substantial increase in the number of nursing homes, while the number of hospitals in the United States has declined (Tirrito, 1993). There are more than 1.4 million residents in nursing homes at any point in time (Tirrito), and the lifetime risk of using nursing home services is more than 40% (U.S. Senate Special Committee on Aging, 1991). It is projected that long-term care service demands will continue to grow significantly (Tirrito, 1993; U.S. Senate Special Committee on Aging, 1991; Vladeck, Miller, & Clauser, 1993). Institutions providing long-term care services are now, and are very likely to continue to be, significant players in health care service delivery to the chronically ill. Policy initiatives targeted to influence institutional policies and subsequently to improve or ensure the quality of services residents receive are very likely to continue.

POLICY ISSUES

Identifying Issues

To gain an up-to-the-minute perspective of the institutional policy issues that surround the current care of chronically ill residents, a descriptive study using qualitative methods was designed. A purposive sample of experts in the field of long-term care was selected. Ten experts were interviewed in-depth, using an unstructured interview guide to identify their perspectives regarding major institutional policy issues faced in the delivery of services to chronically ill residents in nursing homes. Common themes and perspectives were identified.

Major institutional policy issues related to the care of the chronically ill that the experts identified for nursing homes today are

1. financial viability of their organizations,
2. quality of care,

3. coordination of care across different health care settings,
4. end of life decisions for residents and families,
5. use of restraints,
6. managing acute illnesses of chronically ill residents,
7. meeting psychosocial needs of residents and families, and
8. meeting employee needs.

The spectrum of institutional policy issues that these experts are managing is wide and complex. The issues are consistent with those identified in the literature. This chapter is an integration of these themes, perspectives, and relevant literature.

Financial Viability

The major overwhelming issue cited by our experts is the pressure to maintain financial viability of their long-term care organizations. The nursing home industry in the United States is heavily financed by public funding. The Medicaid program enacted in 1965 as Title XIX of the Social Security Act provides health insurance coverage for individuals and families with low incomes. Also enacted in 1965 was Title XVIII of the Social Security Act, Medicare, which is the health insurance for the aged. Medicaid (a federal-state program) is the primary funding source, providing almost 45% of nursing home funding, while Medicare (a federal program) provides only 2%, and private insurance only 1%. These percentages translate in 1990 dollars to almost $16 billion for Medicaid, over $1 billion for Medicare, and $21 billion for out-of-pocket expenditures (U. S. Senate Special Committee on Aging, 1991).

Although the dollars spent for long-term care services are impressive, Medicaid funding does not cover the total costs for nursing home care for Medicaid residents. Nursing home providers are constantly struggling with the shortfall from Medicaid. In an effort to cover the shortfall, many organizations cost-shift to private-pay residents, charging private-pay residents more for their care than the actual costs. However, this strategy is inadequate as a long-term strategy and some states have enacted legislation to prevent cost-shifting from private-pay residents to subsidize the care of Medicaid clients. Medicaid funding policies have a major impact on nursing homes because Medicaid comprises a major portion of a nursing home's budget.

The public perceives the other public payer, Medicare, as a major payer for long-term care services. Because nursing home providers in the 1970s and 1980s perceived Medicare as a potential major funding source, they pursued complying with the more stringent documentation and staffing guidelines of the Medicare program to be able to provide services to Medicare residents. However, the cost of implementing Medicare programming has been burdensome for many smaller, less sophisticated nursing homes or small systems of nursing homes. Even today, it is questionable if there is a real cost-benefit of having Medicare-licensed beds if the usage is limited, though it may provide a method for filling Medicaid beds when residents are no longer eligible for Medicare. This is important in regions of the country where there is an excess of nursing home beds.

A major financial viability issue in the 1990s for long-term care providers is the challenge to develop capitated reimbursement for long-term care services. Providers will be forced to develop capitated packages to fit with managed care contracts that control the costs of acute care and primary care services. The experts we interviewed are struggling to develop formulas at this time. To date, capitation rates have not been determined. To explore capitated payment methods for nursing home services, there is willingness within the federal system for providers to propose capitated programs. These alternative plans require regulatory waivers, which are available from the HCFA.

Some nursing home administrators perceive that the answer to their financial viability lies in the development and expansion of subacute units (Molis, 1993; Singleton, 1994; Stahl, 1994). Subacute care has been described as the provision of a variety of medical-surgical, oncological, rehabilitative, and other specialty services in alternative settings for people who no longer need acute care but are too ill to be sent home (Stahl, 1995a). The cost of subacute care is usually 20%–50% less than the cost of care in acute care hospitals. The payment for subacute care is significantly higher than traditional nursing home care; thus many providers are pursuing developing subacute nursing home units. This strategy is not without risks and challenges. There are new nursing home enforcement regulations that became effective on July 1, 1995, new subacute accreditation standards from the Joint Commission of Accreditation of Healthcare Organizations (JCAHO), managed care contracts with aggressive price controls, as well as the need for nurse managers with strong interdisciplinary, personnel, and financial management skills (Stahl, 1995b).

Jumping into the subacute service delivery should be approached with caution. Is it possible that history will repeat itself? Long-term care may find short-term financial benefits in the development of subacute units. Perhaps additional reimbursement obtained from subacute units will provide a short-lived source of revenue, but will it address the long-term financial viability problem? Could we be repeating the history of the 1970s Medicare units, which were to be the answer to financial viability of nursing homes in the 1970s? There are striking similarities. When Medicare patients were introduced into long-term care in the 1970s, they were more acutely ill than the typical nursing home resident. Today subacute residents are more acutely ill than typical long-term residents of the 1990s. Pursuing subacute units as a financial panacea to nursing home financial viability may likely prove to be resource intensive, with limited financial benefit, just as were the Medicare units of the 1970s.

The experts consistently report that acuity and diversity of residents within their long-term care facilities are greater than ever before. They also explain that residents in subacute units that some are forming have even higher levels of acuity. It is interesting that public policies that regulate long-term care apply across all types of residents. The same federal regulations apply to all types of residents within long-term care facilities regardless of their physical or behavioral acuity or where they are located in the facility, for example, a regular nursing home unit, a dementia special care unit, or a subacute unit. This presents remarkable challenges for administrative and clinical staff. Regulations that make sense for long-stay residents, such as team assessment and care planning taking up to 3 weeks, do not make sense for a subacute unit where the average length of stay is 2 or 3 weeks. The absence of specialized regulations to deal with differences in acuity of residents in subacute units or other nursing home units has stimulated establishing professional standards from other standard setting bodies such as JCAHO and the American Health Care Association (Stahl, 1994).

Quality of Care

A major public policy intent from the OBRA 87 legislation was improving nursing home quality of care. A major legislative expectation was that the quality of care for nursing home residents would improve through the mandate that quality assurance and assessment processes be initiated (Department of Health and Human Services, 1991). While many nursing homes had quality assessment activities in place prior to OBRA 87, now most organizations in long-term care have some type of quality assessment structure within their organizations (Miller & Rantz, 1994).

Many facilities have embraced the notion of continuous quality improvement or total quality management (Ceol, 1993; Dennik-Champion, Marino, & Carlson, 1994). Others are focusing on the quality process and measuring outcomes (Braun, 1991; Johnson, 1991; Rantz, 1995a, 1995b). Regardless of the way that quality is approached as a policy initiative within the agency, the leadership of the organization must create a vision and atmosphere for possibilities that may exist for improving the care.

The experts that we interviewed are not hampered by the notion that they are limited in any way to improve the quality of care for their residents. Although they keep finances in mind, they are open to the possibility that there can be changes in care delivery and they attempt to create structures and systems to improve the quality of clinical care. They raise concerns that only isolated facilities have been able to achieve a high level of quality. These isolated facilities, according to our experts, embrace the process of quality improvement and with their staff have been able to move the organizations to improve the quality of care. Although the regulatory intent was certainly to improve care nationwide, and organizations have put structural pieces of quality assurance or assessment in place, sweeping change and improvement in care at the bedside have yet to be nationally achieved.

Another intent of OBRA 87 was to improve the quality of care through use of a comprehensive resident assessment and care planning system. The Minimum Data Set for Resident Assessment and Care Screening (MDS) and the Resident Assessment Protocols (RAPs) were mandated to be used in all nursing homes (Morris et al., 1990). The MDS includes information about physical, social, behavioral, and emotional well-being, and the RAPs are care planning tools that correspond with MDS items to help identify care issues. In addition, HCFA has funded a large demonstration project to develop and test quality indicators and case-mix payment systems using MDS data (Ryther, Zimmerman, & Kelly-Powell, 1994, 1995). This demonstration is in progress and will provide additional quality of care information for providers as results are analyzed.

Coordination of Care across Settings

A major issue raised by the experts and raised repeatedly in the literature is coordinating services for the chronically ill across the health care delivery system (Rantz & Bopp, 1996). Demonstrations of coordinated service delivery systems were funded in the 1970s and 1980s in an attempt to reduce fragmentation of services, control costs, improve access, and improve quality of services for frail elders (Capitman, Haskins, & Bernstein, 1986; Leutz, Abrahams, Greenlick, Kane, & Prottas, 1988; MacAdam et al., 1989). Like many community-dwelling elderly, most nursing home residents have multiple chronic illnesses. Managing those chronic illnesses within the nursing home environment is not always possible. At times, there are acute exacerbations that require services in an acute care setting. Once stabilized, the residents may return to the long-term care setting or potentially to the community setting.

For people with chronic illness, interfacing between acute, institutional, long-term, and community-based services can indeed be a nightmare. Data elements are different from setting to setting, and assessment instruments differ from setting to setting. Medical record components are repeated, organized in different fashions, and not readily shared. The experts that we interviewed in long-term care not only raised the issue of sharing data, but expressed the need to share the same assessment instrument across settings. The duplication of data collection and lack of coordination of care place additional burdens on organizational systems across the various settings and also place additional burdens on chronically ill clients. The chronically ill do not have the energy to repeatedly provide information to health care providers in various settings. This lack of coordination places an undue burden on clients and families, and it places a costly burden on settings that duplicate data collection and record keeping processes. Missing pieces of data can place clients at great risk for adverse effects.

With the experience of long-term care providers using the standardized MDS, perhaps it is time for them to initiate the development of coordinated assessment instruments and data collection methods that would be used for chronically ill clients across *all* care delivery systems. The usual approach for long-term care as an industry has been to wait for regulations to impose policy decisions such as this. Such an initiative could begin without governmental mandate by existing, nationwide, integrated networks of primary care, acute care, and long-term care services. These existing networks of providers could implement integrated data systems and standardized assessment instruments *across* settings in their organizations nationwide. They could conduct pilot work that could be done cooperatively, rather than being imposed by federal legislation. Pilot work could function as role modeling and influence utilization of integrated data systems and assessment instruments across traditional care settings.

End of Life Decisions

A major thrust of the OBRA 87 legislation was to emphasize residents' rights to self-determination and other rights, such as privacy, the freedom from abuse, access to information, communication and visitation, participation in care planning with the right to refuse treatment, personal possessions, and financial affairs (Streim & Katz, 1994). Subsequently in 1991, the federal Patient Self-Determination Act required that all health care agencies that receive federal funding recognize advanced directives. The act made it the responsibility of health care organizations to promote the knowledge and completion of such documents (Cox & Sachs, 1994). Almost all health care delivery organizations are affected: hospitals, nursing homes, health maintenance organizations, and home health care agencies.

Policy issues surrounding end of life decisions have been brought to the forefront in long-term care by these two regulatory initiatives. Prior to these initiatives, agencies were faced with physicians carrying the major burden as they influenced decisions that families and residents with chronic illnesses would make regarding their treatment. These legislative efforts placed the decision-making power with residents, with their families, and with surrogate decision makers who are familiar with each resident's wishes. Placing decision-making power with residents is a major step forward and one that long-term care agencies should embrace to help residents control these major life choices. Regulatory interpretive guidelines used by nursing home surveyors reinforce the rights of residents to participate in decisions about their care, including end of life decisions.

The tenets of these two regulatory initiatives reflect a major philosophical shift in decision making; however, discussion about this shift is absent in the literature. Most of the literature discusses problems of documents being completed adequately, if information has been distributed to residents and families, and focuses on the problems of informed consent (High, 1994; Krynski, Tymchuk, & Ouslander, 1994; Palmer & Nettles-Carlson, 1995). An examination of outcomes and impact of the philosophical shift that decision-making power now rests with residents, their families, and surrogates is missing. Has there been an effect on the overall decision-making ability of clients? Has this philosophy been transferred to other aspects of client decision making, or has it simply stayed within the narrow focus of end of life decision making? The intent of OBRA 87 was that there be greater empowerment of residents surrounding all decisions in their lives, not just end of life decisions.

Through OBRA 87 and the Patient Self-Determination Act, dialogue among health care providers has increased regarding the appropriateness of initiation or the withdrawal of artificial, nutritional support. No longer is inserting a feeding tube an automatic decision that must be made when confronted with a chronic illness that would require artificial nutritional support to continue life (Hodges & Tolle, 1994; Krynski et al., 1994). While specific regulations vary from state to state, residents and families are participating in decisions regarding initiation or withdrawal of tube feedings for the ending of artificial, nutritional support.

Restraints

A major thrust of OBRA 87 was restricting the use of chemical and physical restraints. Although the industry as a whole did not initially embrace these changes, the results of this legislative effort are empirically supported. There has been a significant reduction in the use of psychotropic drugs as chemical restraints, and the use of psychotropic drugs in general has been reduced (Streim & Katz, 1994). The use of physical restraints has been significantly reduced nationwide, and the development of alternatives to the use of physical and chemical restraints has been pursued (Miles & Meyers, 1994; Rantz & McShane, 1994; Werner, Koroknay, Braun, & Cohen-Mansfield, 1994). Research related to the myth that restraints prevent falls or keep residents safe supports discontinuing the use of physical restraints (Ejaz, Jones, & Rose, 1994; Evans & Strumpf, 1990; Tinetti, Liu, & Ginter, 1992; Werner, Cohen-Mansfield, Koroknay, & Braun, 1994).

While progress in reducing restraint use has been made, some chronically ill residents present behaviors that many agencies continue to have problems managing without the use of physical or chemical restraints (Janelli, Kanski, & Neary, 1994). Some of the experts that we interviewed raise this same concern. There appears to be a subset of nursing home residents who are difficult to manage without those alternatives, especially chemical restraints. There is a need for continued research and the development of creative alternatives for this subset of residents. Experts express those needs. They are concerned that they have been unsuccessful at managing this subset of residents without using some physical and/or chemical restraints. In general, there was widespread success for eliminating restraints for the majority of the chronically ill, long-term care population. The chronically mentally ill residents with other chronic physical illnesses are a particular challenge for staff to identify and recommend alternatives to physical and chemical restraints. Many times, chemical interventions are essential to successful clinical management of these residents. Further research and development are needed to establish criteria that can delineate those individuals who may be appropriate for the use of physical or chemical restraints.

Managing Acute Illness of Chronically Ill Residents

The experts agreed that the level of patient acuity is on the rise. Acuity is, though, not a constant, but an ever-changing client state. Chronically ill nursing home residents frequently experience acute illnesses and chronic illness exacerbations. Policy issues related to reimbursement and adequate staffing affect the retention of these individuals in the nursing home. Nursing homes are faced with decisions to treat at the nursing home or hospitalize for treatment. Payer source policies, such as managed care organizations, are encouraging long-term care to maintain these residents at the nursing home and provide higher technical care there. Nursing home providers are faced with the decision of whether to design separate sections of nursing homes to manage those with acute illnesses or to upgrade the overall skill and knowledge of all nursing staff to be able to safely manage chronically ill residents with acute illnesses in the units where they reside.

Upgrading skills of the nursing staff may, in fact, require that nursing homes incorporate gerontological advanced practice nurses (GAPNs) in greater numbers in the care of the institutionalized chronically ill. The value of GAPNs in nursing homes has been demonstrated; hospitalizations for acute illness are reduced while costs do not significantly increase (Buchanan et al., 1989). Governmental and private organizational policy barriers related to the utilization of these providers will need to be broken down. Two barriers are at issue. Federally, there is a problem with funding for an independent APN (nurse practitioner or clinical nurse specialist). For the APN to receive reimbursement for services provided, he or she is required to be employed by a physician or service provider/clinic (Sharp, 1995). The second issue is that states have created barriers to advanced practice by not allowing APNs to practice to their full scope. For example, prescriptive privileges vary from state to state, and APNs do not have any prescriptive privileges in some states.

Another dimension of acute illness care mentioned by the experts is managing residents who are HIV positive. While people with AIDS are predicted to need long-term care services in ever-increasing numbers, there is a reluctance on the part of nursing homes to provide services to this special group (Linsk, Cich, & Cianfrani, 1993; Vladeck, Miller, & Clauser, 1993). Numerous institutional policy issues surrounding these residents include issues of confidentiality among residents, confidentiality with the staff, and confidentiality with community members coming into the facility. Typically, HIV positive residents and those with AIDS need more care than the normal amount of nursing services allocated in nursing homes. Reimbursement for this care has not been addressed consistently by Medicaid programs. Faced with managing the costly care these people require and the complex issues of confidentiality, many providers are hesitant to accept people with AIDS as residents for care in their facilities.

Meeting Employee Needs

Long-term care has been and continues to be chronically plagued with high turnover rates, low wages, and a negative image. Turnover has been a particular problem for nursing assistants, the workers who provide more than 80% of the care of residents (Hawes, 1991). The 1986 IOM study reported 70% to over 100% annual turnover of nursing assistants. More recently in a study of 26 nursing homes, nursing assistant turnover ranged from 15% to 200%, with an average annual rate of 93% (Caudill & Patrick, 1991). In this same study, registered nurse turnover ranged from 11% to 250%, with an average annual rate of 45%. In addition to high turnover, nursing home staff experience lower wages than other health care workers (Gold, 1995) and higher workers' compensation injury rates (Staff, 1995). Nearly one in five nursing home workers is injured every year.

Image of nursing homes and nursing home workers has been a chronic problem. There are public and professional perceptions that employees in long-term care are somehow of poorer quality than their counterparts in other settings. Although there were major efforts made with OBRA 87 regulations to improve the training of employees in an attempt to attract "better" people working in long-term care, the industry continues to be plagued by a nagging negative image. Part of the image problem can be traced to inadequate Medicaid reimbursement rates and, subsequently, lower salaries of employees. Home health agencies and hospitals pay significantly higher wages than long-term care agencies (Gold, 1995). There is a trend toward higher wages for certified nursing assistants, but registered nurses in long-term care earn an average of 20% less than their counterparts in hospitals. However, licensed practical nurse wages are similar across settings (Gold, 1995).

Image, wage, injury, and turnover problems create challenges to administrators and other managers in long-term care agencies. They must create positive working environments and personnel practices to attract and maintain a good workforce in their agencies. Additionally, they must be proactive in influencing public policies that affect reimbursement to enhance funding available for competitive wages and in supporting staffing levels needed to provide care.

Determining the adequacy of staffing has been another source of controversy. The OBRA 87 regulations established minimum registered nurse staffing requirements. There are advocacy groups and professionals who believe these regulations did not go far enough (Francese & Mohler, 1994). They believe it is critical to increase the registered nurse staff in long-term care. These concerns are not simply a desire for more professionals to practice in these settings. Clinical outcomes research has demonstrated that quality of care and patient outcomes are positively related to registered nurse staffing in nursing homes (Braun, 1991; Institute of Medicine, 1986; Munroe, 1990). Undoubtedly, recruiting and retaining well-qualified registered nurses in long-term care is critical to the care that chronically ill residents receive in these agencies.

To affect recruitment and retention, wages are not the only issue that needs to be addressed. Job satisfaction needs to be understood better. In one study, the most highly ranked sources of dissatisfaction for nurses working in long-term care are an excessive workload, poor staff cohesiveness, poor staffing, and poor working relations with administrators (Carr & Kazanowski, 1994). It is critical that these issues be addressed to assure successful recruitment and retention. Perhaps it is time, once again, to nationally address the issue of increasing the regulations requiring more registered nurses in long-term care. One such national effort that may contribute toward this end is another study undertaken by the IOM on the adequacy of nursing staff in hospitals and nursing homes and the relationship of staffing to quality of care. This study is under way (Maas, Buckwalter, & Specht, 1995). It is expected that results will support increasing the numbers of registered nurses working in our nation's nursing homes.

OBRA 87 did provide increased access of chronically ill nursing home residents to APNs by providing reimbursement for monthly nursing home visits to APNs (nurse practitioners or clinical nurse specialists), who practice in conjunction with physicians. However, utilization of these nursing professionals varies considerably across the United States, and reimbursement for APN services when not practicing in conjunction with physicians is needed. OBRA 87 also opened the door for improved nursing assistant training. It was anticipated that improved training would result in improved retention and improved quality of care. Obviously turnover rates over 100% would not indicate that the long-term care industry is affecting retention through additional training. One legislative intent was to improve the quality of the employees and to improve care. It is uncertain if those outcomes have indeed been realized. In the opinions of the experts that we interviewed, their assessment is that these intents of the legislation have not been met.

CONCLUSION

In the last 4 decades, institutional long-term care has been substantially influenced by federal, state, and organizational policy decisions. Though there have been significant changes within this aspect of care delivery, it is obvious that the intents of all of the initiatives have *not* been realized fully. Professional nurses must become involved in not only the implementation of policy decisions but in the efforts to influence and shape policy decisions affecting the care of institutionalized chronically ill *before* they are made. Only through involvement of professional nurses in greater numbers can the intents to improve quality of care for these residents be achieved.

REFERENCES

Braun, B. I. (1991). The effect of nursing home quality on patient outcome. *Journal of the American Geriatrics Society, 39,* 329–338.

Buchanan, J. L., Arnold, S. B., Bell, R. M., Witsberger, C., Kane, R. L., & Garrard, J. (1989). *The financial impact of nursing home-based geriatric nurse practitioners: An evaluation of the Mountain States Health Corporation GNP project.* Santa Monica, CA: Rand Corporation.

Capitman, J. A., Haskins, B., & Bernstein, J. (1986). Case management approaches in coordinated community-oriented long-term care demonstrations. *Gerontologist, 26*(4), 398–404.

Carr, K. K., & Kazanowski, M. K. (1994). Factors affecting job satisfaction of nurses who work in long-term care. *Journal of Advanced Nursing, 19,* 878–883.

Caudill, M. E., & Patrick, M. (1991). Costing nurse turnover in nursing homes. *Nursing Management, 22*(11), 61–64.

Ceol, D. W. (1993). Total quality management: Orchestrating the changes in long term care. *Provider, 19*(9), 34–38, 40, 43–48.

Cox, D. M., & Sachs, G. A. (1994). Advance directives and the patient self-determination act. *Clinics in Geriatric Nursing, 10*(3), 431–443.

Dennik-Champion, G., Marino, S., & Carlson, J. M. (1994). Transforming quality assurance activities to a quality improvement program. In T. V. Miller & M. J. Rantz (Eds.), *Quality assurance for long-term care* (pp. I:20–I:25). Gaithersburg, MD: Aspen.

Department of Health and Human Services, Health Care Financing Administration. (1991). 42 C. F. R. §§ 431 *et seq.* 56 *Fed. Reg.*, 48,826–48,878.

Ejaz, F. K., Jones, J. A., & Rose, M. S. (1994). Falls among nursing home residents: An examination of incident reports before and after restraint reduction programs. *Journal of the American Geriatrics Society, 42,* 960–964.

Evans, L. K., & Strumpf, N. E. (1990). Myths about elder restraint. *Image: Journal of Nursing Scholarship, 22*(2), 124–128.

Francese, T., & Mohler, M. (1994). Long-term care nurse staffing requirements: Has OBRA really helped? *Geriatric Nursing, 15*(3), 139–141.

Gold, M. F. (1995). Bridging the salary gap in long-term care. *Provider, 21*(4), 43–48.

Hawes, C. (1991). The Institute of Medicine study: Improving the quality of nursing home care. In P. R. Katz, R. L. Kane, & M. D. Mezey (Eds.), *Advances in long-term care.* New York: Springer.

High, D. M. (1994). Surrogate decision making: Who will make decisions for me when I can't? *Clinics in Geriatric Nursing, 10*(3), 445–462.

Hodges, M. O., & Tolle, S. W. (1994). Tube-feeding decisions in the elderly. *Clinics in Geriatric Nursing, 10*(3), 475–489.

Institute of Medicine. (1986). *Improving the quality of care in nursing homes.* Washington, DC: National Academy Press.

Janelli, L. M., Kanski, G. W., & Neary, M. A. (1994). Physical restraints: Has OBRA made a difference? *Journal of Gerontological Nursing, 20*(6), 17–21.

Johnson, J. (1991). Quality assurance: Team approach. *Provider, 17*(5) 16–18, 21–22.

Kane, R. K. (1988). Assessing quality in nursing homes. *Clinics in Geriatric Medicine, 4*(3), 655–666.

Krynski, M. D., Tymchuk, A. J., & Ouslander, J. G. (1994). How informed can consent be? New light on comprehension among elderly people making decisions about enteral tube feeding. *Gerontologist, 34*(1), 34–46.

Leutz, A., Abrahams, M. A., Greenlick, M., Kane, R., & Prottas, J. (1988). Targeting expanded care to the aged: Early SHMO experience. *Gerontologist, 28*(1), 4–17.

Linsk, N. L., Cich, P. J., & Cianfrani, L. (1993). The AIDS epidemic: Challenges for nursing homes. *Journal of Gerontological Nursing, 19*(1), 11–22.

Maas, M., Buckwalter, K., & Specht, J. (1995). *IOM report: Nursing staff and quality of care in nursing homes.* A report prepared for the Institute of Medicine, University of Iowa College of Nursing.

MacAdam, M., Capitman, J., Yee, D., Prottas, J., Leutz, W., & Westwater, D. (1989). Case management for frail elders: The Robert Wood Johnson Foundation's program for hospital initiatives in long-term care. *Gerontologist, 29*(6), 737–744.

Migdail, K. J. (1992). Nursing home reform: Five years later. *Journal of American Health Policy*, 2(5), 41–46.

Miles, S. H., & Meyers, R. (1994). Untying the elderly. *Clinics in Geriatric Nursing, 10*(3), 513–525.

Miller, T. V., & Rantz, M. J. (1994). *Quality assurance for long-term care.* Gaithersburg, MD: Aspen.

Molis, D. B. (1993). New directions in long-term care: The emergence of subacute care. *Provider, 19*(8), 22–24, 30–32.

Morris, J. N., Hawes, C., Fries, B. E., Phillips, C. D., Mor, V., Katz, S., Murphy, K., Drugovich, M. L., & Friedlob, A. S. (1990). Designing the national resident assessment instrument for nursing homes. *Gerontologist, 30*(3), 293–307.

Munroe, D. J. (1990). The influence of registered nurse staffing on the quality of nursing home care. *Research in Nursing & Health, 13,* 263–270.

Palmer, N. B., & Nettles-Carlson, B. (1995). The prevalence of advance directives: Lessons from a nursing home. *Nurse Practitioner, 20*(2), 7–8, 13, 17–19.

Rantz, M. J. (1995a). Quality measurement in nursing: Where are we now? *Journal of Nursing Care Quality, 9*(2), 1–7.

Rantz, M. J. (1995b). Nursing quality measurement: A review of nursing studies. Washington, DC: American Nurses Publishing.

Rantz, M. J., & Bopp, K. (1996). Issues in care, design, & implementation from acute, long-term care, & community-based settings. In E. Cohen (Ed.), *Nursing case management for the 21st century* (pp. 181–188). St. Louis: Mosley Year Book.

Rantz, M. J., & McShane, R. (1994). Nursing home staff perception of behavior disturbance and management of confused residents. *Applied Nursing Research, 7*(3), 132–140.

Ryther, B. J., Zimmerman, D., & Kelly-Powell, M. (1994). Using resident assessment data in quality monitoring. In T. V. Miller & M. J. Rantz (Eds.), *Quality assurance for long-term care* (pp. I:26–I:28). Gaithersburg, MD: Aspen.

Ryther, B. J., Zimmerman, D., & Kelly-Powell, M. (1995). Update on using resident assessment data in quality monitoring. In T. V. Miller & M. J. Rantz (Eds.), *Quality assurance for long-term care* (pp. I:28–I:29). Gaithersburg, MD: Aspen.

Sharp, N. (1995). Medicaid reimbursement introduced for all NPs and CNSs. *Nursing Management, 26*(7), 88–91.

Singleton, G. W. (1994, May). Transitioning to subacute: The keys to success. *Nursing Homes, 43*(4), 16–18.

Staff. (1995). Nursing home workers run high risk of injury. *Health Facilities Management, 8*(6), 7–8.

Stahl, D. A. (1994). Subacute care: The future of health care. *Nursing Management, 25*(10), 34, 36, 38–40.

Stahl, D. A. (1995a). Managed care and subacute care: A partnership of choice. *Nursing Management, 26*(1), 17–19.

Stahl, D. A. (1995b). Subacute care: 1995 leadership challenges for SNFs. *Nursing Management, 26*(3), 17–19.

Streim, J. E., & Katz, I. R. (1994). Federal regulations and the care of patients with dementia in the nursing home. *Medical Clinics of North America, 78*(4), 895–909.

Tinetti, M. E., Liu, W. L., & Ginter, S. F. (1992). Mechanical restraint use and fall-related injuries among residents of skilled nursing facilities. *Annals of Internal Medicine, 116*(5), 369–374.

Tirrito, T. (1993). Reimbursement mechanisms and their impact upon nursing home patients. In J. A. Toner, L. M. Tepper, & B. Greenfield (Eds.), *Long-term care: Management, scope and practical issues* (pp. 42–53). Philadelphia: Charles Press.

U.S. Senate Special Committee on Aging, the American Association of Retired Persons, the Federal Council on the Aging, and the U.S. Administration on Aging. (1991). *Aging America* (DHHS Publication No. FCOA 91-28001). Washington, DC: U.S. Department of Health and Human Services.

Vladeck, B. C., Miller, N. A., & Clauser, S. B. (1993). The changing face of long-term care. *Health Care Financing Review, 14*(4), 5–23.

Werner, P., Cohen-Mansfield, J., Koroknay, V., & Braun, J. (1994). The impact of a restraint-reduction program on nursing home residents. *Geriatric Nursing, 15*(3), 142–146.

Werner, P., Koroknay, V., Braun, J., & Cohen-Mansfield, J. (1994). Individualized care alternatives used in the process of removing physical restraints in the nursing home. *Journal of the American Geriatrics Society, 42,* 312–325.

Zimmerman, D. R. (1991). Impact of new regulations and data sources on nursing home quality of care. In *Mechanisms of quality in long-term care.* New York: NLN Press.

Epilogue: Policy Issues Related to Accessible Health Care for Older Adults

Elizabeth A. Swanson

The authors of this book have touched on many implications for nursing in meeting the health needs of chronically ill elders. They have discussed the chronically ill elderly from the various vantage points of their areas of expertise, but an overarching theme emerges across the chapters: *accessible health care.* This theme can be defined as care that is available, acceptable, and affordable. Throughout the book, the authors have identified the cultural, economic, political, and social factors that have a profound effect on accessible health care for the older adult. For example, Dimond, Catanzaro, and Lorensen refer to the health care issues faced by older women due to patterns of socioeconomic and gender stratification within American society. Approaching the issue of accessible health care from an economic perspective, Powers as well as Corbin and Cherry in their separate chapters identify the decreasing availability of material and human resources in health care, which affects older adults' capacity to care for themselves effectively.

Additional documentation regarding the degree of accessibility of care services for older Americans is found in *Old age in the 21st century: A report to the Assistant Secretary for Aging, U.S. Department of Health and Human Services,* prepared by the National Academy on Aging (1994). This report brings into question the extent to which satisfactory health care services will be available to older Americans, based on its finding that current services for elders in the United States are insufficient and of poor quality, and many providers of the services are inadequately educated and trained. The report continues to state that when excellent quality services do exist, individuals and their family members may not be aware of them, may be unaware of their own needs for such services, or are unable to arrange for the services. This lack of knowledge and insight to health care needs suggests the need for increasing the awareness of health professionals to the importance of assessing the requirements of older adults comprehensively, arranging and coordinating services, and evaluating their effectiveness.

A report from the Federal Council on the Aging (1994), *The need for home and community-based long-term care: A rural perspective,* also questions the availability of long-term care and other health services. As a part of their summary of major findings, the authors conclude that in general, home and community-based care for rural elders and their families are often less comprehensive, offered less frequently, and not as accessible as comparable services in urban settings. The report also indicated that while there are some excellent resources available for long-term care in rural areas, the projected need for these services is going to increase dramatically after the year 2000 (Federal Council on the Aging).

Notably, both the National Academy on Aging report and the Federal Council on the Aging report suggest that health professionals give concerted attention to designing service models and strategies for long-term care. Clearly, the design process can and should heed the documented importance of home and community-based care in providing health care for the older adult. The relevance of these services can be noted from different perspectives. For example, Morse and Dellasega, in their chapter on qualitative research, note that 90% of older persons, including most of the chronically ill, live at home. In the book *Improving health policy and management,* Wiener and Hanley (1992) support this fact and purport that older adults want to stay in their homes and be independent. Not only are the wishes of the older adult important, but other benefits exist. Remaining at home rather than in an institution often translates into a better quality of life, a reduction in the use of institutional care and related costs, an increased number of options for the individual and family members, and a delay of further decline due to meeting existent health care needs (Federal Council on the Aging, 1994). Thus within this context, it is significant to examine methods to enhance the provision of long-term care services to the older adult.

The provision of long-term care services is controlled by the Medicare and Medicaid systems. However, these two systems support primarily medical and institutional care. Consideration needs to be given to developing a long-term care system that supports a range of care choices and alternatives, such as those suggested by the authors of this book and by the federal reports previously mentioned.

One service option might be the establishment of interdisciplinary teams designed to work with older adults and their families in the planning, coordinating, and acquisition of comprehensive care. Advanced nurse practitioners working as a part of this interdisciplinary team within an agency setting could work directly with the older adult and family and serve as the key coordinator of health care services. Nurses could work very effectively within this model because they are knowledgeable of the cultures of the different agencies of care, they have the skills to integrate the work of multiple providers of care and to facilitate decision making, and they can seek out funding to cover the cost of the care. In addition, the nurse could implement the mechanism for defining the standards against which programs of care need to be implemented and evaluated. Steps should be taken by policy makers to ensure that at least every county has an agency of this nature available to it (National Academy on Aging, 1994). The role of the agency would not be to provide the direct services, but to facilitate through the interdisciplinary team the planning, coordinating, and arranging of comprehensive care.

Financial incentives need to be developed and implemented to acknowledge the contribution of the team and reward it for the effort spent in the planning, coordinating, and arranging of care, as no direct provision of care would occur. Since the financial incentive is tied to the team function, team leadership and composition would have to be constructed carefully to ensure third-party payment from Medicare, Medicaid, Blue Cross/Blue Shield, or any other commercial insurance program.

Another service option for older adults is the community-based, nurse-managed center, such as the Chai Health Center described by Corbin and Cherry. It is through such nurse-managed clinics that underserved individuals can have their health needs met successfully. For example, information and referral services can be provided to individuals, as can health-promotion programs to improve the older adults' overall well-being, prevent health problems, and reduce health care costs. But again the question of reimbursement arises. Who will be paid for the provision of direct care, and will health-promotion services be covered under any type of payment system? Payment authorizations for these nonphysician practitioners should be at least at the level of 85% of the Medicare physician fee schedule. With the presence of a multidisciplinary team, consideration also needs to be given that services delivered by the team members or the head of the team be billed by someone licensed to provide those services. In addition, policy makers also need to consider covering disease preventive measures, mental health, and dental health services. If payment for health-promotion activities is not forthcoming, we as health professionals can at least acknowledge the appropriateness of these health-promotion and disease preventive activities for the older adult. With this acknowledgement, health professionals could assist elders to plan activities that serve to enhance the quality of their life.

Changes in the payment source for in-home services also need to be made. Insurance programs for long-term care are beginning to be developed across the nation. This insurance needs to pay for in-home services, as the demand for such services will increase sharply. Ideally, suggests Kenneth Thorpe (1994), long-term care insurance should provide coverage for both in-home assistance and nursing home care. As discussed previously, this approach can be cost-effective, since in-home services are usually less expensive than nursing home care. This payment approach may be a more useful financing source for older adults in the future, as opposed to present-day older individuals, as Thorpe remarks that group policies are being sold to large employee groups at very reasonable rates. Regardless of the source of funding for services of this nature, older adults need to be informed better about the costs of long-term care services, or they will not seek out additional sources of funding when the opportunity exists.

The previous brief suggestions focus on the "formal" care services that currently exist or could be enhanced by introducing changes in the approach to service delivery or by implementing policy changes. But the preference of older persons for community-based services enabling them to stay at home compels us also to acknowledge the role of informal caregiving. This epilogue has also mentioned the need for family members to be involved in the care of the older adult, and it has suggested how nurses could work together with the older adult and family members to meet the comprehensive health needs of the older individual. One could conclude, as Walker, Pratt, and Eddy (1995) have, that there is a need for the intensification of the interface between formal and informal caregivers. Yet it is critical that health professionals and policy makers understand that formal services do not take the place of services provided by family. Wiener and Hanley (1992) contended that the provision of formal in-home services to care for older persons does not result in a decrease of the services provided by the family members, but rather in an increase in the degree to which the total needs of the individual are met. This contention is particularly significant, given recent attempts by the federal government to decrease the availability of health care services to those elders with families (Hooyman, 1990).

The community-based clinic structure can play a critical role in the meshing of the formal and informal approaches. Educational programs can be offered to train family caregivers and equip them with the skills and abilities to provide direct care to their chronically ill family members. Support groups can be organized that are designed to help alleviate the individual stress of family caregivers.

An interface of services for elders can also occur between the family member(s) and the health care providers of the long-term care institution. Partnerships can be developed between family members and the staff of the long-term care facilities. Research on the effectiveness of such an approach is currently being conducted at the University of Iowa College of Nursing. At several long-term care study sites, family-staff caregiving partnerships have been developed that allow the care needs of the residents with dementia to be met by both the formal and informal caregivers. Agreements are developed between the staff and the family members as to the care duties each party will be responsible for providing. In particular, family members are responsible for providing information about the resident, providing care to meet the resident's basic activities of daily living needs, or providing care to meet instrumental living needs of the resident.

As with other efforts to change the care delivery approach, this type of initiative has encountered barriers, and certain elements within the long-term care environment need to be changed to facilitate the implementation of shared caregiving.

1. Policies need to be implemented that require adequate staff in long-term care facilities, including the availability of a team of professional staff. This suggestion is consistent with the Institute of Medicine's (IOM) report (1986), which calls for enhancements in the staff mix in nursing homes and recommends the use of geriatric nurse specialists and geriatric nurse practitioners for leadership and direct care positions in long-term care.

2. Family members need to be welcomed when they visit, and communications with the staff need to be conducted on a regular basis. One

way in which the communication can be improved is to involve the family members in the care conferences. This approach would provide both family and staff with a forum to clarify expectations, share information, resolve conflict, and facilitate the interface of the formal and informal systems of care.

3. Staff and administrators of long-term care facilities need to revisit the purpose, structure, and content of existing care conferences to actively involve the family members of their residents. This revisiting may call for policy changes within their facility or organization.

Certainly, other resources will exist in the 21st century that health professionals have not had available to them until most recently. Technological innovations such as the fax machine, e-mail, interactive audio and video, and telemedicine have a vast capability to enhance the access to health care for all individuals. Technological applications can be used to enhance communication across the professions and to less populated sections of the country. Discussions of medical examinations and evaluations, psychosocial assessments, and family conferences can be conducted over the information superhighway. Teleradiology is advancing and becoming more common as a diagnostic tool in practices (Fickenscher & Lagerwey-Voorman, 1992). Using strategies of this nature enhances the knowledge and expertise of health care providers while reducing the need to have direct on-site observation and assessment. These strategies can be adapted within a clinic site, and protocols can be developed to empower the nurse to conduct the on-site assessment and forward the relevant data to a physician colleague at a major, secondary, or tertiary care facility. Care approaches like these can be an excellent method of providing high quality service that is allocated more efficiently.

In summary, data indicate there will be increasing numbers of older adults and family members who will require a range of long-term care services in the 21st century. Nurses can play a significant role in helping establish policies and procedures that expand the availability, accessibility, and affordability of health care services to the older adult. For example, community-based clinics and informal caregiving approaches can permit the chronically ill older adult to remain in the community and live independently. These approaches can afford the individuals involved a higher quality of life, reduce health care costs, and serve to maximize the care options that are available to the older adults and their family members.

This volume of *Advances in Gerontological Nursing* has attempted to identify some of the issues, concerns, and possible approaches to address the health care needs of chronically ill elders, both now and in the coming decades. The most important implication of this compilation of information is that as a health profession, nursing needs to plan and act now to meet those needs. As the Federal Council on the Aging (1994) suggests, the choices will only become more costly and the response more pressing with time.

REFERENCES

Federal Council on the Aging. (1994, August). *The need for home and community-based care: A rural perspective* (Issue Brief, Vol. 1, No. 1). Washington, DC: Author.

Fickenscher, K., & Lagerwey-Voorman, M. (1992). An overview of rural health care. In S. M. Shortell & U. E. Reinhardt (Eds.), *Improving health policy and management: Nine critical research issues for the 1990s* (pp. 111–149). Ann Arbor, MI: Health Administration Press.

Hooyman, N. (1990). Women as caregivers: Implications for social welfare policy and practice. In D. Biegel & A. Blum (Eds.), *Aging and caregiving: Theory, research and practice* (pp. 221–241). Beverly Hills, CA: Sage.

Institute of Medicine. (1986). *Improving the quality of care in nursing homes.* Washington, DC: National Academy Press.

National Academy on Aging. (1994). *Old age in the 21st century: A report to the Assistant Secretary for Aging, U.S. Department of Health and Human Services.* Washington, DC: Author.

Thorpe, K. E. (1994). Health care cost containment: Results and lessons from the past 20 years. In S. M. Shortell & U. E. Reinhardt (Eds.), *Improving health policy and management: Nine critical research issues for the 1990s* (pp. 227–274). Ann Arbor, MI: Health Administration Press.

Walker, A. J., Pratt, C. C., & Eddy, L. (1995). Informal caregiving to aging family members. *Family Relations, 44,* 402–411.

Wiener, J. M., & Hanley, R. J. (1992). Caring for the disabled elderly: There's no place like home. In S. M. Shortell & U. E. Reinhardt (Eds.), *Improving health policy and management: Nine critical research issues for the 1990s* (pp. 75–110). Ann Arbor, MI: Health Administration Press.

Index

DATE DUE
